Pathogen Inactivation: The Penultimate Paradigm Shift

AABB PRESS

Other related publications available from the AABB:

Technical Manual, 16th edition
Edited by John D. Roback, MD, PhD;
Martha Rae Combs, MT(ASCP)SBB; Brenda J. Grossman, MD; and
Christopher Hillyer, MD

The AABB Press publishes books and CDs on many topics of interest to those in the blood banking, transfusion medicine, and cellular therapy fields.

To purchase books or to inquire about other book services, including chapter reprints and large-quantity sales, please contact our sales department:

- 866.222.2498 (within the United States)
- +1 301.215.6499 (outside the United States)
- +1 301.951.7150 (fax)
- www.aabb.org>Bookstore

AABB customer service representatives are available by telephone from 8:30 am to 5:00 pm ET, Monday through Friday, excluding holidays.

Pathogen Inactivation: The Penultimate Paradigm Shift

Editors

James P. AuBuchon, MD, FCAP, FRCP(Edin)
President and Chief Executive Officer
Puget Sound Blood Center
Professor of Medicine (Hematology) and of Laboratory Medicine
University of Washington
Seattle, Washington

Christopher V. Prowse, MA, DPhil, FRCPathol
Research Director
Scottish National Blood Transfusion Service, Edinburgh
Honorary Senior Lecturer
College of Medicine and Veterinary Medicine
Edinburgh University
Edinburgh, Scotland

AABB Press
Bethesda, Maryland
2010

Mention of specific products or equipment by contributors to this AABB Press publication does not represent an endorsement of such products by the AABB Press nor does it necessarily indicate a preference for those products over other similar competitive products.

AABB Press authors are requested to comply with a conflict of interest policy that includes disclosure of relationships with commercial firms. A copy of the policy is located at http://www.aabb.org.

Efforts are made to have publications of the AABB Press consistent in regard to acceptable practices. However, for several reasons, they may not be. First, as new developments in the practice of blood banking occur, changes may be recommended to the AABB *Standards for Blood Banks and Transfusion Services.* It is not possible, however, to revise each publication at the time such a change is adopted. Thus, it is essential that the most recent edition of the *Standards* be consulted as a reference in regard to current acceptable practices. Second, the views expressed in this publication represent the opinions of authors. The publication of this book does not constitute an endorsement by the AABB Press of any view expressed herein, and the AABB Press expressly disclaims any liability arising from any inaccuracy or misstatement.

AABB
8101 Glenbrook Road
Bethesda, Maryland 20814-2749

ISBN NO. 978-1-56395-309-5
Printed in the United States

Library of Congress Cataloging-in-Publication Data

Pathogen inactivation : the penultimate paradigm shift / editors, James P. AuBuchon, Christopher V. Prowse.

p. ; cm.

Includes bibliographical references and index.

ISBN 978-1-56395-309-5

1. Blood—Collection and preservation. 2. Disinfection and disinfectants. 3. Bloodborne infections—Prevention. I. AuBuchon, James P. II. Prowse, Christopher V. III. AABB.

[DNLM: 1. Blood Transfusion—adverse effects. 2. Blood Platelets—microbiology. 3. Blood-Borne Pathogens. 4. Communicable Disease Control—methods. WB 356]

RM172.P38 2010

615'.39—dc22

2010037645

AABB Press Editorial Board

Contributors

Georges Andreu, MD, PhD
Institut National de la Transfusion
Sanguine, Paris, France

Celso Bianco, MD
America's Blood Centers
Washington, District of Columbia

Jose A. Cancelas, MD, PhD
Hoxworth Blood Center
University of Cincinnati Academic
Health Center
Cincinnati, Ohio

Joy A. Cavagnaro, PhD
Access BIO, LC
Boyce, Virginia

Jean-Pierre Cazenave, MD, PhD
Etablissement Français du Sang Alsace
Strasbourg, France

Sigrid Cherrier-De Wilde, MD
Centre Hospitalier
Luxembourg, Luxembourg

Joan Cid, MD, PhD
Institut d'Investigacions Biomèdiques
August Pi i Sunyé
Barcelona, Spain

Roger Y. Dodd, PhD
American Red Cross
Rockville, Maryland

Øystein Flesland MD, PhD
Norwegian Knowledge Centre
for the Health Services
Oslo, Norway

Peter Hellstern, MD
Institute of Hemostaseology and
Transfusion Medicine
Academic City Hospital Ludwigshafen
Ludwigshafen, Germany

Reinhard Henschler, MD, PhD
German Red Cross Blood
Transfusion Service
Baden-Wuerttemberg-Hessen
Frankfurt/Main, Germany

Bernard Horowitz, PhD
Horowitz Consultants, LLC
Key Biscayne, Florida

Hervé Isola
Etablissement Français du Sang Alsace
Strasbourg, France

Louis M. Katz, MD
Mississippi Valley Regional
Blood Center
Davenport, Iowa

Daniel Kientz, MD
Etablissement Français du Sang Alsace
Strasbourg, France

Harvey G. Klein, MD
National Institutes of Health
Bethesda, Maryland

Richard M. Lewis, PhD
Access BIO, LC
Boyce, Virginia

Miguel Lozano, MD, PhD
Institut d'Investigacions Biomèdiques
August Pi i Sunyé
Barcelona, Spain

Jeffrey McCullough, MD
Institute for Engineering in Medicine
University of Minnesota
Medical School
Minneapolis, Minnesota

Olga Mikulich, MD, PhD, MRCPI
St James's Hospital
Dublin, Ireland

Markus M. Mueller, MD
German Red Cross Blood
Transfusion Service
Baden-Wuerttemberg-Hessen
Frankfurt/Main, Germany

William G. Murphy, MD, FRCPEdin, FRCPath
University College
Dublin, Ireland

Jean Claude Osselaer, MD, JD
Mont-Godinne Blood
Transfusion Establishment
Yvoir, Belgium

Christopher V. Prowse, DPhil, FRCPath
Scottish National Blood
Transfusion Service
Edinburgh, Scotland
United Kingdom

Erhard Seifried, MD, PhD
German Red Cross Blood
Transfusion Service
Baden-Wuerttemberg-Hessen
Frankfurt/Main, Germany

Bjarte G. Solheim, MD, PhD, MHA
Institute of Immunology
Oslo University Hospital—
Rikshospitalet
University of Oslo
Oslo, Norway

Chantal Waller, MD
Etablissement Français du Sang Alsace
Strasbourg, France

Table of Contents

Current Status of Technologies for Components

Practical Experience of Implementation

Preface

Like any other medical intervention, the transfusion of blood components is expected by clinician and patient alike to be safe and effective. Countless millions of patients owe their lives to the effectiveness of modern hemotherapy. Although concerns have been aired about the effect of storage lesions, and there remains room for improving the efficacy of transfusion, modern medicine has taken good advantage of the benefits of transfusion.

The risks of transfusion have attracted considerable attention over the years, however. First it was hepatitis—recognized early as coming in at least two varieties—that raised concern. Then it was a peculiar new disease caused by a (then) "new" type of virus (retrovirus) that resulted in devastating effects for unfortunate patients: human immunodeficiency virus (HIV). Thankfully, each of these threats to blood safety has been met with the development of effective donor education and screening tools and the deployment of sensitive and specific detection techniques. No longer do blood bankers watch the evening television news fearful of hearing of yet another report of the failure to deliver the viral safety that is expected of their efforts. Public expressions of concern about transmission of variant Creutzfeldt-Jakob disease serve to remind us of the importance of our mission. For the most part, the public, believing the blood supply is safe, has moved on to other concerns. And it *is* safe—but not assuredly so.

Although we recognize that a "zero-risk" blood supply is an unattainable dream, we are grateful for the reduction in the risks associated with identified pathogens. However, as our scientific abilities improve, we recognize that the number of pathogens that may be transmitted from human to human—and possibly through transfusion—is astoundingly large. NNV, the next new virus, is certainly out there and more a risk than we might like to admit. Last year an AABB task force reviewed and published, in a special supplement of *TRANSFUSION*, advice on 68 separate pathogens and how they might adversely affect the safety of transfusion. Some questions arise:

- Can we, and will we, react to the documented arrival of the next pathogen threat with a new test quickly enough?
- Can we afford to keep adding (single, pathogen-specific) test after test when we *do* recognize the risk?
- Will manufacturers be there to "rescue" us from the precipice?
- Will we devote resources to "middle-range" threats that are not as large as HIV but nevertheless cause some morbidity or mortality?

Then we also have those threats that we have not been able to deal with definitively. The most notable of these is bacteria contaminating platelets. Graft-vs-host disease has an antidote in irradiation, to be sure, but we know from hemovigilance data that this prevention is not always applied to patients at risk, and it carries with it undesirable expenses, complexities, and complications.

In this imperfect world, pathogen-inactivation techniques have been sought as a panacea. As detailed in this text, nothing comes without a price—not only monetary but, ironically, also in terms of questioned safety or efficacy. The cost per life saved or infection averted for known pathogens will be astronomical, as measures already in place have successfully reduced these risks to very low levels.[1,2] The real potential, as emphasized in Chapters 1 and 16, is likely to be seen in addressing the next new virus and in reducing the risk that has been least effectively addressed by testing to date—bacterial contamination of platelets. For plasma and platelets today, and, hopefully, for red cells in the not-too-distant future, we have the capability of virtually "waving a magic wand" and removing (or substantially reducing) the scourges that, like specters, have so shaped our practice of transfusion medicine in the last quarter-century. The advent and broad acceptance of pathogen inactivation for all labile blood components would truly be the proverbial paradigm shift.

A variety of technologies have been developed for use with labile blood components (see table). Licensure of these is more advanced in Europe than in North America. Indeed, as described in Chapter 17, of 20 European blood collectors, 18 are using pathogen-inactivated plasma in one or more forms, and nine have implemented use of pathogen-inactivated platelets, although not necessarily in all blood banks or for all patients.

For this monograph, we have been fortunate to obtain contributions from a cross-section of international authorities with experi-

Status of Current Technologies

Component	Company	Technique	Status
Red Blood Cells	Cerus	S303	Phase II clinical trials
	CaridianBCT	Riboflavin + UV	Phase I clinical trials
	Vitex	Inactine	Abandoned
Platelets	Cerus	Amotosalen + UV	CE marked (2002)
	CaridianBCT	Riboflavin + UV	CE marked (2007)
	Macopharma	UV	Phase III clinical trials
Plasma	Cerus	Amotosalen + UV	CE marked (2006)
	CaridianBCT	Riboflavin + UV	CE marked (2008)
	Macopharma	Methylene blue + light	CE marked (2000)
	Octapharma	Solvent/detergent	Licensed* (>1991) (pools)
	VIPS; Colombier, Switzerland	Solvent/detergent	CE marked (2009) (single donor/minipools)

*OctaPlas is licensed as a prescription medicine rather than a medical device in Europe (1991/1992 in Germany, France, Norway, and Belgium; 1998 in the United Kingdom).
UV = ultraviolet (light); CE = Conformité Européenne.
Single donor methylene blue, and pooled solvent detergent, treated plasma are also produced under licence by Grifols S.A., Barcelona, Spain and by the Bordeaux CRTS in France, respectively.

ence in the field of investigating and applying pathogen-inactivation techniques. We have attempted to focus on clinical trials and practical implementations completed to date by a number of "early adopters" in order to give those not currently using these techniques the best possible view of how they will fit into one's current system and how they provide what patients need. Although some authors have performed research studies for the manufacturers of these techniques, we have attempted to provide the most independent of voices to allow the reader assurance of objectivity.

We leave it to the readers to assess these data in their own regulatory and health-care environments and to determine whether we are yet at the threshold of a new paradigm. It is our belief that these techniques, while not fulfilling our complete wish list, have much to offer recipients, with the simultaneous assumption of remarkably little risk.

So, is this the future of transfusion medicine? Perhaps, but we await with hope the final paradigm shift—that of the generation of cellular blood components and a multifunctional plasma substitute via ex-vivo manufacture. These techniques, while clearly still in their infancy, have the potential to transform "blood banking" from a system of medical care based on a community's altruism and an uncontrollable "raw material" source to a pharmaceutical manufacturing endeavor that can generate products indistinguishable from their biologic templates, free of infectious and immunologic risks, without storage-induced changes, and reliably available. Knowing that this hope remains ephemeral for now, we look to pathogen inactivation of labile blood components as the *penultimate* paradigm shift.

James P. AuBuchon, MD
Chris V. Prowse, DPhil
Editors

References

1. Janssen MP, van der Poel CL, Buskens E, et al. Costs and benefits of bacterial culturing and pathogen reduction in the Netherlands. Transfusion 2006;46:956-65.
2. Custer B, Agapova M, Martinez RH. The cost-effectiveness of pathogen reduction technology as assessed using a multiple risk reduction model. Transfusion 2010 May 24 (epub ahead of print).

About the Editors

James P. AuBuchon, MD, FCAP, FRCP(Edin), attended the University of Michigan for undergraduate work in cellular biology and medical training before entering the field of pathology. He completed an anatomic and clinical pathology residency at the University of Wisconsin and was a senior staff fellow in the Department of Transfusion Medicine at the National Institutes of Health for 2 years. Subsequently, he worked in the American Red Cross Blood Services system for 6 years before spending 18 years at Dartmouth-Hitchcock Medical Center as the medical director of the blood bank and transfusion service and then as the E. Elizabeth French Professor and chair of pathology and professor of medicine. He relocated to Seattle, WA, to become the president and chief executive officer of Puget Sound Blood Center in September 2009. Currently, Dr. AuBuchon is the president-elect of the AABB; he is also the past-chair of the Biomedical Excellence for Safer Transfusion (BEST) Collaborative and the former chair of the Transfusion Medicine Resource Committee of the College of American Pathologists.

Christopher V. Prowse, MA, DPhil, FRCPath0l, obtained both his first degree and his doctorate from Oxford University, in biochemistry and on the structural aspects of coagulation proteins, respectively. In the subsequent 34 years, he has worked in various research and operational posts within the Scottish National Blood Transfusion Service in Edinburgh and Glasgow and was appointed as research director in 1999. His research interests have included hemostasis, monoclonal antibodies, blood components and their processing (including pathogen-inactivation technologies), emerging infections (particularly variant Creutzfeldt-Jakob disease and the establishment of nucleic acid testing for viruses), and cellular therapies. He has been a member of the British Blood Transfusion Society Council, The BEST Collaborative, the Hemaquebec Safety Advisory Committee, the UK Prion Working Group, The Medical

Committee of the World Federation of Haemophilia, and the Transfusion-Transmitted Infection Committee of the International Society for Blood Transfusion. Dr. Prowse chairs the UK Standing Advisory Committee on Blood Components; runs a master of science course on transfusion, transplantation, and tissue banking in Edinburgh; and is an examiner in hematology and transfusion for the Royal College of Pathology.

In: AuBuchon JP, Prowse CV, eds.
Pathogen Inactivation: The Penultimate Paradigm Shift
Bethesda, MD: AABB Press, 2010

1

Pathogen Inactivation: Rationale and Some History

HARVEY G. KLEIN, MD

There are known knowns. These are things we know that we know. There are known unknowns. That is to say there are things that we know we don't know. But there are also unknown unknowns. There are things we don't know we don't know.

—Donald Rumsfeld, US Secretary of Defense
Department of Defense news briefing
February 12, 2002

SINCE THE 17TH CENTURY AND THE FIRST TRANSfusion of blood from sheep to man, the history of blood transfusion has been marked by high expectations and unanticipated complications. The complications have often spurred technical adjustments that have resulted

Harvey G. Klein, MD, Department of Transfusion Medicine, Clinical Center, National Institutes of Health, Bethesda, Maryland

Disclaimer: This article was written in a personal capacity and does not necessarily represent the opinions or endorsement of the National Institutes of Health, the Department of Health and Human Services, or the Federal Government.

The author has disclosed no conflicts of interest.

in impressive advances in lifesaving supportive care. Much of this history involves recognition of unexpected blood-borne pathogens and efforts to reduce the risk of their transmission by transfusion. The first successful human transfusion, using a syringe to transfer blood from donor to recipient, is attributed to the English obstetrician James Blundell in 1818. Unfortunately, the patient died. In his report, Blundell cautioned that transfusion should be reserved for patients in extremis.[1] Mortality in Blundell's published series approached 50%, but probably not as a result of transfusion-transmitted infection. His patients and those of many of his successors received fresh blood that was unlikely to be subject to bacterial growth; malaria was not endemic in England; and Blundell's patients often did not live long enough to experience the effects of chronic viral infection, should these even have been suspected long before Bassi proposed the germ theory of disease.[2]

The era of modern transfusion medicine dates to the early 20th century, with the identification of the major blood groups by Landsteiner in 1901.[3] Subsequent use of the agglutination technique for compatibility testing improved blood safety dramatically and expanded its use, although recognition of the immunologic diversity of red cells and sophisticated crossmatching had to await the discovery of the direct antiglobulin (Coombs) test almost 50 years later.[4] In the early 20th century, blood was transfused directly from donor to patient via arteriovenous anastamosis, a technique perfected by Alexis Carrell and for which he was awarded the Nobel Prize in 1912. One unexpected consequence of fresh blood transfusion was transmission of *Treponema pallidum*, the agent responsible for syphilis, from donor to recipient (and occasionally from recipient to donor). By 1937, syphilis was the most commonly recognized disease transmitted by transfusion.[5]

Three measures likely contributed to the virtual eradication of syphilis as a transfusion-transmitted infection in the United States: 1) the striking efficacy of penicillin in reducing prevalent cases among potential donors; 2) the development of anticoagulant-preservative solutions and refrigerated storage by Rous and Turner,[6] because spirochetes fail to thrive at refrigerator temperatures; and 3) the introduction of donor screening by a serologic test for syphilis in 1938 and its requirement by federal regulation in 1945.[7] These three strategies—improving the health status of the donor, reducing the pathogens in the product, and screening for known transmissible pathogens—have become cornerstone interventions for reducing the infectious risks of transfusion. Of some interest is the absence of any donor screening question regarding syphilis or risk activity related to syphilis. Perhaps these were more modest times. The last recorded case of syphilis attributed to transfusion in the United States more than 40 years ago was likely transmitted by room-temperature-stored platelets collected from a volunteer donor.[8] One lesson to be gleaned from the syphilis experience is that, when available, pathogen inactivation is generally a more reliable intervention than are donor selection and screening strategies. At the very least, one could say that refrigeration as a "half-way technology" for pathogen reduction, though not really introduced for that purpose but for maintaining red cell viability, added a belt to the existing suspenders.

A further bane of early transfusion practice was the severe, even fatal, febrile transfusion reaction that commonly resulted from contamination of reusable flasks and bottles by bacteria and bacterial products. Margaret Pittman reviewed this literature in 1953 and emphasized that bacterial contamination of blood was largely unreported.[9] Febrile reactions that had complicated virtually every early transfusion had been reduced to 10% or fewer by the 1950s, and fatal reactions, probably caused by bacteria in whole blood units, were estimated at somewhere between 1 in 10,000 and 14 in 10,000 transfusions. At about the same time, the plastic blood container was being developed by Fenton and Walter.[10] Within a decade, the advent of sterile, interconnected disposable plastic blood bags and universal refrigeration of stored blood had all but erased this problem from the medical radar screen.[10] Bacteria would not re-emerge as a recognized transfusion risk for almost 25 years, when the risk of sepsis from platelet components stored at room temperature was "rediscovered" as the most common transfusion-transmitted infectious risk.[11,12]

By the middle of the 20th century, transfusions had been implicated in the transmission of viral illness, although the scope of the problem was not widely appreciated. As noted perceptively by Paul Beeson[13] in the first description of posttransfusion hepatitis:

> *It seems highly probable that they [hepatitis transmissions] may be occurring not infrequently but are not being recognized. If one were not aware of the fact that jaundice may follow inoculation with homologous serum or plasma after a long latent period, one would be unlikely to attach any significance*

to a history of transfusion three months previous to onset of a patient's illness.

By this time one might say that there were "known knowns"—that certain bacteria, viruses, and parasites could be transmitted by transfusion. There were also "known unknowns"—agents that might be spread by blood exposure but not documented to be transfusion transmitted and diseases that seemed to be related to transfusion but for which no agent had been identified; non-A, non-B hepatitis is an example of the latter. In addition, there were "unknown unknowns." The idea that some "new" infectious diseases might suddenly appear in pandemic form and pose great risk to transfusion recipients was not of great concern to most physicians in the 1970s; AIDS changed that. A selection of known transfusion-transmissible viral agents is given in Table 1-1.

Current Risk Abatement Model

Until recently, the approach to the risk of pathogen transmission through blood transfusion has relied almost exclusively on a combination of donor education, selection of low-risk donors (volunteer, nonremunerated), donor screening by direct questioning regarding risk behavior, testing for select causative agents, consulting of lists of previously deferred donors, meticulous examination and preparation of the phlebotomy site, discarding components in quarantine or inventory if evidence of donor exposure or illness is reported after donation, and donor tracing and notification when instances of disease transmission were detected.[14] This strategy has proven effective. In developed countries, the risk of transfusion-transmitted viral infection is now so low that it cannot be measured directly; mathematical modeling is required to estimate the residual risk.[15] Calculated residual risks of transfusion-transmitted viruses in repeat US blood donors approximate 1:2,135,000 for human immunodeficiency virus (HIV), 1:1,935,000 for hepatitis C virus (HCV), 1:144,000 for hepatitis B virus (HBV), and 1:641,000 for human T-cell lymphotropic virus, types I and II (HTLV-I/II).[16] Risks are estimated to be even lower in Europe.[17] The system of safeguards is somewhat less effective, and certainly less efficient, for interdicting bacterial and parasitic infections. Yet blood is safer than it has ever been. So what is the problem?

Table 1-1. Selected Human Blood-Borne Viral Infectious Agents

Viral Pathogen	Family	Genome	Enveloped	Size (nm)	Transmitted by: Cellular Products	Transmitted by: Plasma Products
Human immunodeficiency virus, types 1 and 2	Retro	ss-RNA	+	80-100	Yes	Yes
Human T-cell leukemia, types I and II	Retro	ss-RNA	+	80-100	Yes	No
Hepatitis A virus	Picorna	ss-RNA	–	27-32	Yes	Yes
Hepatitis B virus	Hepadna	ds-DNA	+	40-48	Yes	Yes
Hepatitis C virus	Toga	ss-RNA	+	40-50	Yes	Yes
Hepatitis delta virus	Delta	ss-RNA	+	36	Yes	Yes
Hepatitis E virus	Calci	ss-RNA	–	35-39	Yes	Yes
Hepatitis G virus	Flavi	ss-RNA	+	40-60	Yes	Yes
West Nile virus	Flavi	ss-RNA	+	40-60	Yes	Yes
Human erythrovirus B19	Parvo	ss-DNA	–	18-26	Yes	Yes
TT virus	Circo	ss-DNA	+	30-50	Yes	Yes
Epstein-Barr virus	Herpes	ds-DNA	+	120-220	Yes	Yes
Cytomegalovirus	Herpes	ds-DNA	+	130-200	Yes	No
Human herpes 8 virus	Herpes	ds-DNA	+	120-200	Yes	No

ss = single stranded; ds= double stranded; + = presence of a lipid envelope; – = no lipid envelope.

Understanding the issues begins with considering the current paradigm. The cornerstone of blood component safety today rests on a strategy of surveillance and testing. The first screening test used in the United States was really a surrogate assay—the serologic test for syphilis, which was introduced in 1938. It was not particularly effective then and is probably close to useless today. However, once introduced, tests intended to improve blood safety are not easily changed. With the recognition of HBV, screening assays based first on agar gel diffusion and later on counterelectrophoresis were developed and deployed in the early 1970s. These were not very sensitive or specific, nor were they easily automated or highly regulated. It is often underappreciated that test development is not static, whether it involves serology or direct viral detection. Testing evolves over years or decades after initial licensure. The costs evolve as well. The advent of the radioimmunoassay and enzyme-linked immunosorbent assay (ELISA) improved the ease and reliability of HBV screening dramatically, but they also revealed that the majority of posttransfusion hepatitis cases were caused by some other agent or agents.[18] What followed was a decade of surrogate testing with assays for elevated liver enzymes or for the antibody to hepatitis B core antigen (HBc).[19,20] Not until 1989 was HCV discovered and a specific test for antibody to HCV developed.[21] An estimated 4.8 million transfusion-transmitted HCV infections occurred between 1970 and 1990; on the basis of a 20% incidence of severe outcomes, these might have resulted in more than 700,000 cases of cirrhosis in the United States.[22]

Several weaknesses in the current surveillance and testing strategy have been widely recognized. Infections slip through the seronegative "window," the interval between donor infection and virus detection. With current sensitive nucleic-acid-based assays, the windows for HCV, HIV, and even HBV are now reduced to a few weeks or less. There is always the risk of laboratory error, erroneous release of quarantined units, viral variants that go undetected by current assays, donors who are seronegative carriers with low levels of virus, or even apparently immune, occult carriers, but these probably account for a small number of infections.[23]

The real risk is the "emerging agent," the prototype for which was HIV. If a new agent—with a long silent period, ready transmission by transfusion, and potential for secondary spread—were to infect the blood supply tomorrow, recipients of blood components would be almost as vulnerable now as they were in the early 1980s before

HIV was identified as the causative agent of AIDS. The risk in San Francisco of receiving an infectious unit before the first case of transfusion-associated AIDS was recognized has been estimated in excess of 1%.[24] One might think that such an occurrence is unique. However, the recent experience with West Nile virus (WNV) was not so dissimilar. Fortunately, on the one hand, the clinical consequences of WNV were sufficiently acute to bring it to national attention soon after its introduction into the United States, and on the other, the majority of the infections were subclinical and apparently without long-term consequence. There was no secondary spread. The disease was not invariably fatal. And finally, although a screening test was developed and licensed in record time, a research diagnostic test was already available when WNV was recognized in the United States (unlike the situation with HIV). Despite these attributes that led to containment relatively quickly, still hundreds to thousands of transfusion-transmitted infections likely occurred before screening was put in place. In 2002 alone, before screening could be implemented, 23 transfusion-transmitted clinical cases were confirmed, seven of whom died of the disease; these numbers are generally considered a gross underestimate of the true problem. Increasing human contact with animal species, international travel, and changes in the environment guarantee that similar epidemics will occur. The only questions are When? and What will they look like?

Surveillance and screening is necessarily a reactive strategy. Delay is inevitable. As Harvey Alter has emphasized, years may elapse from the discovery of an etiologic agent to implementation of a licensed test.[21] For HBV, that interval was 30 years; for non-A, non-B hepatitis/HCV, 15 years; and for HIV, WNV, *Trypanosoma cruzi*, and bacteria, 3, 4, 5, and 18 years, respectively. There are now a dozen or more screening tests in the armamentarium if tests for specific recipient populations [cytomegalovirus (CMV), Epstein-Barr virus (EBV)] and those in development and likely to be added (malaria) are included. The assays vary both in their quality and effectiveness. The concept of regional testing has been introduced with WNV and is being considered for babesiosis given the geographical differences in prevalence of the causative agent.[25] The costs associated with the process of deciding on and introducing each new test—and the modifications to licensed information systems, especially with regional testing algorithms—are not usually calculated in the cost of blood safety. Furthermore, the value of even recently introduced screening tests, such as the serologic assay for *T. cruzi*, in reducing disease burden has not been established. Numerous additional pathogens are on the horizon. Testing for most recognized emerging or re-emerging agents would result in a greatly reduced blood supply (discussed further below), and attempting to perform scientifically valid risk/benefit analyses on proposed screening tests for all possible pathogens is probably an exercise in futility.

Measures introduced to increase blood safety may have the unintended consequence of decreasing blood availability. Availability is, after all, a safety issue too. Results from demographic studies indicate that certain potential donor groups or donor sites present an unacceptable risk of disease transmission. For example, blood collectors no longer schedule mobile drives at prisons or institutions for the mentally impaired because of the recognized high prevalence of transfusion-transmissible viruses in their residents. Few would argue the risk/benefit analysis of these exclusions. More questionable are the temporary exclusions of soldiers exposed to multiple tick bites at Fort Chaffee, Arkansas; the 1-year deferral for service men and women returning from Iraq; or civilian donors excluded because of travel to Mexico and parts of the Caribbean. A study of 116,165 persons who presented to a regional blood center during the year 2000 indicated that 13.6% were deferred at presentation. Long-term deferral, for example for travel to a malarial area, accounted for 21% of these.[26] More troublesome, though not as large, are donor deferrals resulting from false-positive results of infectious disease screening tests. Disease-marker-reactive donations represented 0.9% of donation deferrals in the study above. This problem has been recognized since the introduction of serologic tests for syphilis. However, over the past 15 years the introduction of new screening tests and testing technologies has resulted in numerous deferrals for "questionable" test results and in either complex re-entry algorithms or no approved method to requalify such donors. Surrogate tests used for screening have proved particularly troublesome.[27] However, even specific tests result in inappropriate deferrals. Several million donors now fall into this category of deferral for false-positive or unconfirmed test results. The costs of counseling and medical referral—not to mention the toll on the donor, the donor's family, and intimate contacts—have yet to be calculated.

A Different Paradigm—Pathogen Removal/Inactivation

There is another model of risk reduction. To begin to understand it, it will be useful to consider that the United States supports a dual system of blood collection. Whereas blood and its components are collected from volunteers, most plasma for fractionation is collected from paid donors by commercial firms. As a result of the AIDS epidemic and the almost universal HIV infection of patients with severe hemophilia treated with pooled-plasma-derived clotting factors, commercial plasma fractionators took determined efforts to introduce methods to remove and inactivate pathogens in the plasma pools. This was a stepwise process. Plasma pools were already treated by a process (Cohn fractionation) involving multiple steps of precipitation, physical separation, and changes in pH, temperature ionic strength, and ethanol concentration gradients. Some pathogen reduction occurred after different steps of precipitation and filtration in the fractionation process; proteins isolated later in the schematic were generally safer from infectious agents.[28] The albumin and globulin fractions proved extremely safe, particularly regarding transmission of hepatitis viruses and HIV. However, the process was not infallible, and deviations from proper processing have resulted in disease transmission. Also of note is that some of the most important plasma protein derivatives are separated early in the fractionation process and do not reap the benefits of added layers of fractionation and processing.

In 1985, when viral inactivation of specific plasma protein clotting fractions was introduced, more than 90% of hemophiliacs were already infected with HCV and HIV. Pasteurization had been used effectively to inactivate viruses in albumin fractions stabilized with small-chain fatty acids from as early as 1948.[29] Other proteins, especially clotting factors, denatured during the pasteurization process unless additional stabilizers were added. As a result of the AIDS experience, manufacturers modified their procedures. Stabilizers were subsequently added and removed by diafiltration or chromatography later in the process. Terminal heat inactivation of lyophilized clotting factors required modification of temperature and processing time. Dry heat treatment of lyophilized clotting factors at 60 to 68 C for 24 to 72 hours did not prevent transmission of HBV and HCV.[30] Increasing the dry heat temperature to 80 C for 72 hours did destroy these viruses, although nonenveloped viruses, especially hepatitis A virus (HAV) and human parvovirus B19, were not completely inactivated. Vapor heating further improved viral kill. Additional manipulation of temperature and pH improved yields of different proteins. The pasteurization process evolved over several years to meet the needs of the users.

Use of organic solvents and detergents in the processing of coagulation factors inactivates lipid-enveloped viruses such as HIV, HBV, HCV, HTLV, EBV, CMV, and herpes 6, 7, and 8 viruses.[31] Incorporation of a virucidal detergent and solvent [the solvent 1% tri-n-butyl phosphate (TNBP) and the detergent 1% Triton X-100 for 4 hours at 30 C) disrupts the lipid envelope and prevents the virus from binding to cells and replicating. The TNBP is removed by oil extraction, and Triton X-100 is removed by chromatographic adsorption. Plasma protein concentrates have been made from solvent/detergent (SD)-treated plasma, and equivalent Fresh Frozen Plasma (FFP) has been licensed in the United States and Europe. As with the heat-inactivated coagulation factors, SD technology does not inactivate the nonenveloped viruses. SD treatment also results in some loss of integral plasma proteins such as α-2 antiplasmin and protein S.[31] Even though this process was far from perfect, it added a layer of safety to the production of plasma fractions.

Nanofiltration, also known as viral filtration, uses sieving or size exclusion to remove infectious agents.[32] Most viruses range in size from approximately 20 to 200 nm (see Table 1-1), and the typical nanofilter has a pore size of 15 to 40 nm. Nanofiltration has proven effective in removing a wide range of viruses, including some nonenveloped viruses, and may even remove viruses smaller than the filter pore size. Proposed mechanisms for the removal of these small agents include viral adsorption at the charged membrane surface, aggregation of the smaller viruses, or association of the viruses with cellular components.[33] Nanofiltration typically results in a 4- to 6-log_{10} removal of most viruses, with 90% to 95% recovery of protein activity. Prion removal from plasma has been achieved when a 10- to 35-nm pore size is used; however, the amount of prion removed depends on the degree of aggregation of the prions. Extensive experience with nanofiltration has not yielded evidence of protein alteration or neoantigen formation.

The details of commercial pathogen inactivation procedures remain proprietary. What is known is that US regulatory authorities require that at least two different methods of removal or inactivation be applied to create an inactivated pooled fractionation product.

Many currently licensed plasma-derived coagulation factors and immunoglobulins that are subjected to heat, pasteurization, and/or SD treatment are also nanofiltered. All classes of plasma protein fractions, such as antithrombin, C-1 inhibitor, protein C, fibrinogen, and ceruloplasmin, have been nanofiltered without apparent change in the protein characteristics.

The paradigm of pathogen inactivation that has been pioneered by the commercial fractionation industry has been hugely successful. No instances of transmission of HIV, HBV, or HCV have been reported from appropriately manufactured products since 1987.[34] As WNV emerged as a transfusion threat in the United States, no transmissions were documented from the plasma fractions. It is only fair to point out that pathogen reduction of plasma for fractionation has not eliminated many of the screening strategies and tests introduced for the collection of whole blood, and these play a role in ensuring safety. Although the cost of inactivated products has been substantially higher than that of the earlier untreated products and recovery of proteins has been reduced, this strategy has been accepted worldwide. It would be considered immoral to return to the previous generation of untreated products.

The Way Forward

A great deal has been learned from a quarter of a century's experience with pathogen reduction of plasma fractions, and these lessons should be applied to blood components. The potency of the plasma proteins in the fractions has been well maintained, and despite some losses during processing, quality and quantity are satisfactory. No significant toxicity from the additives has been encountered over many patient-years of observation. There has been little evidence of immunogenicity from the treated products. Reducing viral agents by 3 to 4 $\log_{10}$ will not reliably interdict disease transmission, but a reduction of 6 to 7 $\log_{10}$ is quite effective.

Why have the not-for-profit blood collectors been slow to embrace the pathogen-reduction model? The answers are probably related to science, to culture, to regulatory hurdles, and to cost—and not necessarily in that order. The blood supply is currently perceived as very safe, and risk/benefit models do not generally include calculations of possible new agents, the "unknown unknowns." Surveillance and screening have proved successful, albeit slow, in dealing with emerging pathogens. There is as yet no single method to inactivate pathogens in all blood components, so the logistics of applying different technologies to the various components seems formidable. Moreover, no method appears capable of inactivating all of the recognized agents: small, tightly-packaged viruses such as HAV are difficult to inactivate; viruses that achieve extremely high titer, such as parvovirus B19, exceed the limits of current inactivation methods; and the problems posed by spores in the vegetative state and prions have yet to be solved. Finally there is the issue of cost. Even if a safe and robust technology can be applied to blood components, no one expects this to be cost neutral, even with the elimination of some current testing costs, avoidance of future tests, and the likely avoidance of the need to irradiate select blood components. However, as discussed previously, many of the ongoing costs of the testing paradigm go unacknowledged.

The foregoing points should not minimize the differences and the challenges of moving toward pathogen inactivation. Inactivating cellular components is far different from inactivating plasma pools. Cells may be more fragile, and small modifications may be more likely to affect function or to result in alloimmunization. Single-donor plasma units might contain higher titers of virus than are found in the plasma pools, and many proteins, not just a single assayed factor, need to be preserved. Treating individual components in plastic bags is a far cry from treating large volumes of plasma in fractionation tanks by adding a step or two to the process. There is substantial concern that pathogen inactivation might expose millions of patients—including gravid women, immunosuppressed patients, and premature infants—to chemicals or altered cells, the long-term effects of which cannot be predicted. The definitive determination of safety comes only after years of clinical use. Finally, if an early technology is developed, will blood services and governments adopt it? Notwithstanding this concern, several European countries are moving ahead with implementation; France, Belgium, and Germany have long used pathogen-reduced plasma and are in the process of introducing such technologies to treat platelet concentrates despite the cost. There is reason for caution but not for unreasonable delay, and happily the process of embracing the new paradigm is underway.[35-37]

The two strategies are not mutually exclusive for ensuring the safest, most effective blood transfusions. It is unlikely that many of the current screening procedures and tests will soon be eliminated by the introduction of pathogen inactivation, but some will be retired over time and new tests and donor questions will probably not need to be added. No single pathogen inactivation method will likely be effective for every class of agent and for every blood component. Some combination of techniques that remove and inactivate infectious agents will almost certainly be needed, at least initially. It is important to recognize that, as with the plasma fractions, the first inactivation techniques will not be the last. Waiting until the ideal system has been developed truly makes the perfect the enemy of the good. These technologies are generally expensive and have the potential to escalate the cost of blood. However, if potent pathogen inactivation techniques that preserve blood function and do not evidence some new toxic risk can be created, the developed world, which often embraces the myth of zero-risk transfusion, will likely adopt them. For the developing world, in which low-risk blood donors are at a premium and elegant testing methods often not feasible, a good but not perfect pathogen reduction method, especially if relatively inexpensive and easy to implement, could save millions of lives.

References

1. Blundell J. Observations on the transfusion of blood. Lancet 1828-1829;2: 321-4.
2. Kyle RA, Shampo MA. Agostino Bassi (biography). JAMA 1979;241:1584.
3. Landsteiner K. Über Agglutinationserscheinungen normalen menschlichen Blutes. Klin Wochenschr 1901;14:1132.
4. Coombs RRA, Mourant AE, Race RR. A new test for the detection of weak and "incomplete" Rh agglutinins. Br J Exp Path 1945;26:255.
5. Kilduffe RA, DeBakey M. The blood bank and the technique and therapeutics of transfusion. St. Louis, MO: CV Mosby, 1942.
6. Rous P, Turner JR. Preservation of living red blood corpuscles in vitro. II. The transfusion of kept cells. J Exp Med 1914;23:219.
7. Minimum requirements: Citrated whole blood (human). Bethesda, MD: National Institute of Health, December 9, 1945.
8. Chambers RW, Foley HT, Schmidt PJ. Transmission of syphilis by fresh blood components. Transfusion 1969;9:32-4.
9. Pittman M. A study of bacteria implicated in transfusion reactions and of bacteria isolated from blood products. J Lab Clin Med 1953;42:273-88.
10. Walter CW. Invention and development of the blood bag. Vox Sang 1984; 47;318-24.

11. Braine HG, Kickler TS, Charache P, et al. Bacterial sepsis secondary to platelet transfusion: An adverse effect of extended storage at room temperature. Transfusion 1986;26:391-3.
12. Benjamin RJ, Kline L, Dy BA, et al. Bacterial contamination of whole-blood-derived platelets: The introduction of sample diversion and prestorage pooling with culture testing in the American Red Cross. Transfusion 2008;48: 2348-55.
13. Beeson PB. Jaundice occurring one to four months after transfusion of blood or plasma—report of seven cases. JAMA 1943;121:1332.
14. Busch M, Chamberland M, Epstein J, et al. Oversight and monitoring of blood safety in the United States. Vox Sang 1999;77:67-76.
15. Wang B, Schreiber GB, Glynn SA, et al for the Retrovirus Epidemiology Donor Study. Does prevalence of transfusion-transmissible viral infection reflect corresponding incidence in United States blood donors? Transfusion 2005; 45:1089-96.
16. Alter HJ, Holland PV, Morrow AG, et al. Clinical and serological analysis of transfusion-associated hepatitis. Lancet 1975;2:838-41.
17. Dodd RY, Notari EP, Stramer SL. Current prevalence and incidence of infectious disease markers and estimated window-period risk in the American Red Cross blood donor population. Transfusion 2002;42:975-9.
18. Pillonel J, Laperche S. Trends in residual risk of transfusion transmitted viral infections (HIV, HCV, HBV) in France between 1992 and 2002 and impact of viral genome screening (nucleic acid testing). Transfus Clin Biol 2004;11:81-6.
19. Koziol DE, Holland PV, Alling DW, et al. Antibody to hepatitis B core antigen as a paradoxical marker for non-A, non-B hepatitis agents in donated blood. Ann Intern Med 1986;104:488-95.
20. Aach RD, Szmuness W, Mosley JW, et al. Serum alanine aminotransferase of donors in relation to the risk of non-A,non-B hepatitis in recipients: The transfusion-transmitted viruses study. N Engl J Med 1981;304:989-94.
21. Alter HJ, Purcell RH, Shih JW, et al. Detection of antibody to hepatitis C virus in prospectively followed transfusion recipients with acute and chronic non-A, non-B hepatitis. N Engl J Med 1989;321:1494-500.
22. Alter HJ. Pathogen reduction: A precautionary principle paradigm. Transfus Med Rev 2008;22:97-102.
23. Candotti D, Allain JP. Transfusion transmitted hepatits B virus infection. J Hepatol 2009;51:798-809.
24. Busch MP, Young MJ, Samson SM, et al. Risk of human immunodeficiency virus (HIV) transmission by blood transfusions before the implementation of HIV-1 antibody screening. The Transfusion Safety Study Group. Transfusion 1991;31:4-11.
25. Kleinman SH, Williams JD, Robertson G, et al. West Nile virus testing experience in 2007: Evaluation of different criteria for triggering individual-donation nucleic acid testing. Transfusion 2009;49:1160-70.
26. Custer B, Johnson ES, Sullivan SD, et al. Quantifying losses to the donated blood supply due to donor deferral and miscollection. Transfusion 2004;44: 1417-26.

27. Linden JV, Gregorio DI, Kalish RI. An estimate of blood donor eligibility in the general population. Vox Sang 1988;54:96-100.
28. Burdick MD, Pifat DY, Petteway Jr SR, Cai K. Clearance of prions during plasma protein manufacture. Transfus Med Rev 2006;20:57-62.
29. Kingdon HS, Lundblad RL. An adventure in biotechnology: The development of haemophilia A therapeutics—from whole blood transfusion to recombinant DNA to gene therapy. Biotechnol Appl Biochem 2002;35:141-8.
30. Mariani G, Ghirardini A, Mandelli F, et al. Heated clotting factors and seroconversion for human immunodeficiency virus in three hemophilic patients. Ann Intern Med 1987;107:113.
31. Prince AM, Horowitz B, Brotman B. Sterilization of hepatitis and HTLV-III viruses by exposure to tri(n-butyl)phosphate and sodium cholate. Lancet 1986; 1:706-10.
32. Klein HG, Dodd RY, Dzik WH, et al. Current status of solvent/detergent-treated frozen plasma. Transfusion 1998;38:102-7.
33. Yokoyama T, Murai K, Murozuka T, et al. Removal of small non-enveloped viruses by nanofiltration. Vox Sang 2004;86:225-9.
34. Centers for Disease Control and Prevention. Blood safety monitoring among persons with bleeding disorders—United States, May 1998-June 2002. MMWR Morb Mortal Wkly Rep 2003;51:1152-4.
35. Osselaer JC, Cazenave JP, Lambermont M, et al. An active haemovigilance programme characterizing the safety profile of 7437 platelet transfusions prepared with amotosalen photochemical treatment. Vox Sang 2008;94:315-23.
36. Williamson LM, Cardigan R, Prowse CV. Methylene blue-treated fresh-frozen plasma: What is its contribution to blood safety? Transfusion 2003;43:1322-9.
37. Ambruso DR, Thurman G, Marschner S, Goodrich RP. Lack of antibody formation to platelet neoantigens after transfusion of riboflavin and ultraviolet light-treated platelet concentrates. Transfusion 2009;49:2631-6.

In: AuBuchon JP, Prowse CV, eds.
Pathogen Inactivation: The Penultimate Paradigm Shift
Bethesda, MD: AABB Press, 2010

2

The Targets

ROGER Y. DODD, PHD

THE INHERENT PROMISE OF PATHOGEN INACTIVATION is to eliminate infectivity and certain other biologically adverse threats from blood components. The purpose of this chapter is to examine this expectation in the context of the real world. Four broad, interacting issues have to be considered. First, the infectious agents in blood components may be present with varying titers and differ in their susceptibility to the inactivation processes. Second, the process of routine donation testing significantly reduces the residual titers of infectious agents in those products that are nonreactive and qualify for transfusion. Third, the physical chemistry of inactivation

Roger Y. Dodd, PhD, Vice President, Research and Development, American Red Cross, Holland Laboratory, Rockville, Maryland

The author has disclosed no conflicts of interest.

processes inevitably results in a progressive decay of infectivity rather than a definitive elimination of all infectivity. Finally, the processes available to date have some damaging effects on the blood components themselves, so any process reflects a balance between inactivation of pathogens and preservation of blood function. It is for these reasons that regulatory agencies, at least in the United States, refer to the process as "pathogen reduction" over "pathogen inactivation."

Infectious Agents in Blood for Transfusion

A number of infectious agents are well-known contaminants of blood components and are already subject to significant (but not complete) control by a combination of donor selection and laboratory testing. These include hepatitis B and C viruses (HBV and HCV), the human immunodeficiency viruses (HIV-1 and HIV-2), and the human lymphotropic retroviruses (HTLV-I and HTLV-II). In the United States and Canada, nucleic acid testing (NAT) for West Nile virus (WNV) is routinely performed. Regarding bacteria, testing for syphilis is routine, and automated culture is performed to detect bacterial contamination of apheresis platelets. In some countries testing has also been introduced for antibodies to *Trypanosoma cruzi*, the agent of Chagas disease. Selective testing may be performed according to patient needs, particularly for cytomegalovirus (CMV). In some parts of the world, NAT is also performed for the B19 parvovirus (B19V). In considering these agents as targets for pathogen reduction, it is appropriate to consider whether the process would be expected to supplement or to displace the testing.

Another group of agents is known to be transmissible by transfusion but does not have any current test-based intervention. Perhaps malaria is the best-known disease in this category, but consideration has to be given to a number of other agents, including dengue and chikungunya viruses, babesia (at least in some locales), leishmania, and variant Creutzfeldt-Jakob disease (vCJD).

Finally, there is a large group of emerging infections that have, on occasion, been transmitted by blood, or that have properties that suggest their transmissibility by this route. Over 60 such agents were recently described in detail.[1]

Well-Known Transfusion-Transmitted Agents

Perhaps surprisingly, there is relatively little direct information about the infectious titers of even the best-characterized transfusion-transmissible infectious agents. Certainly there are a number of indirect or presumptive measures, but the only explicit infectivity titrations that have been performed on humans were those involving HBV in the 1950s, in which a pool of plasma positive for hepatitis B surface antigen was apparently minimally infectious when as little as 1 mL of a 10^7-fold dilution was administered to a research subject.[2-4] It is reasonable to assume that significantly higher infectivity titers might be present in some individual samples. This finding is compatible with information about the extent to which needle-sticks had been shown to be infectious for HBV (30% to 67% of the time). Understandably, there are no comparable human titration studies for other major transfusion-transmissible infections, but there are a number of potential surrogate measures of infectivity, ranging from observational studies on needle-stick and transfusion exposure to measures of viral genome titers. Experience has shown, for example, that needle-stick injuries involving blood from HCV- and HIV-infected individuals result in infection in about 3% and 0.3% of cases, respectively,[5,6] suggesting that these agents have significantly lower infectivity titers than does HBV. In some cases, animal-model titrations and/or data on infectivity in laboratory culture systems are also available. A recent (2009) review provides extensive discussion of the levels of viral nucleic acids and infectivity levels during varying stages of infection with key transfusion-transmissible viruses.[7]

In summary, measured levels of nucleic acids suggest that, for most transfusion-transmissible viruses, maximal levels are on the order of 10^6 to 10^8 copies per mL, with a potential for considerably higher levels for some viruses, most notably B19V and HBV. Serologic test methods for antibodies will significantly reduce the number of donations with these high levels, but because high titers may be achieved during the ramp-up phase before the appearance of antibodies, they cannot ensure that all high-titer samples are identified. In contrast, tests for nucleic acids (and, where available, viral antigens) will limit the maximum titer among units that are nonreactive in such tests. However, overall and as discussed below, there does not seem to be good correspondence between nucleic acid levels and infectivity titers.

Much is currently known about the levels of viral nucleic acids during the early phases of infection with HBV, HCV, HIV, WNV, and, to a lesser extent, dengue virus.[8-12] However, it is not entirely clear how well these nucleic acid levels equate with infectivity in the context of transfusion. A very conservative assumption would be that one or two genome equivalents are equal to a single infectious dose, but available data do not necessarily support this simple model. Indeed, this is illustrated indirectly by the fact that in early infection, the yield of samples positive only in nucleic acid tests tends to be consistent with window-period models based on measures of doubling time. However, the number of infections detected among blood recipients is usually much lower than that predicted by models based on the concept that 1 or even 10 genome copies per transfused unit would be infectious. Of course, a part of this is due to the inefficiency of detection of transfusion-associated infections, but there is also another line of evidence based on look-back studies. More specifically, using HIV as an example, there have been a number of cases in which look-back has identified transmission of infection from a plasma unit but not from the corresponding red cell component (which would have contained only about 20 mL of plasma).[9]

A recent review of all such observations, in association with animal model studies, has suggested that the best estimate of the ID_{50} (dose that would be expected to infect 50% of recipients) for window-period samples is 6.3 RNA copies for HIV, 7 RNA copies for HCV, and 8.2 DNA copies for HBV, with a probable range of 1 to 100. At the same time, it is noted that there are cases in which components with nondetectable levels of nucleic acids do cause infection as well as cases in which relatively high total levels of nucleic acids have apparently failed to infect a recipient. For each of these disease agents, it is further suggested that the infectious dose for samples collected during the chronic, or set-point, phase is 75- to 100-fold greater, perhaps reflecting the modulating effect of coexisting antibodies on infectivity.[7]

Some information about the minimal infectious dose of WNV may be obtained from breakthrough infections derived from blood donations that are viremic but undetectable in pooled testing. Appropriate use of single-donation testing in times or places with high incidence rates for WNV infection seems to prevent or at least significantly reduce such infections. The 95% detection limit with single-donation testing for WNV is around 10 copies/mL, so presumably an infectious dose might be greater than 200 to 2000 RNA copies. (It is notable that in tissue culture, one plaque-forming unit is equivalent to about 400 copies).

In summary, it appears that current NAT methods do have the capacity to reduce residual levels of key transfusion-transmissible pathogens to the extent that there may be no more than 10^2 to 10^3 infectious doses in a unit of blood, platelets, or plasma. Further, it appears that, in some cases at least, the levels in a red cell concentrate may be below infectious levels. Current data on the efficacy of pathogen-reduction methods clearly suggest that they would be expected to remove such residual levels of infectivity with ease.

Other Viral Agents

A number of other viruses are of actual or potential concern in the context of blood safety. Two arboviruses have attracted considerable attention: dengue virus (a flavivirus) and chikungunya virus (an alphavirus). There are published reports of two clusters of dengue transmission via transfusion,[12-15] along with publications that detail findings of viremic donations from asymptomatic individuals. RNA levels of 10^8 or more copies per mL have been reported, and such high-titer samples are clearly infectious in tissue culture and mosquito models.[12] Similarly, chikungunya virus has emerged rapidly and widely and has been responsible for explosive outbreaks over the past few years. Although transfusion transmission has not been documented, measures to reduce the risk of such an occurrence have been taken in some affected areas.[16-18] Such measures included rapid implementation of NAT, introduction of pathogen-reduction technologies, and cessation of local collection of blood or selected components. Again, very high titers of viral RNA have been found in asymptomatic individuals.

Another virus that has been studied in some detail is B19V. It is the cause of a mild childhood exanthema but may have severe or even fatal outcomes for the fetus if infection is contracted during pregnancy. Additionally, infection can lead to aplastic crisis in individuals with hemolytic disease states. The virus is readily transmitted by transfusion, and levels of viremia can be extremely high—up to 10^{14} copies per mL.[19] However, severe transfusion-transmitted disease has only rarely been reported. Unlike many of the other viruses mentioned, B19V is nonenveloped and appears to be somewhat resistant to at least some inactivation protocols. This is also true of hepatitis A virus, another occasional cause of transfusion-transmitted infection.

There are other viruses that are definitely transfusion transmissible, are usually cell-associated, and tend to be present at low (sometimes essentially undetectable) levels. Some retroviruses (particularly HTLV-I and -II) and a number of herpes viruses, including CMV and human herpes 8 virus, fall into this category.

Finally, it has been learned that, contrary to earlier thinking, there is no predictable pattern for an emerging, transfusion-transmissible virus. It used to be thought that the most likely candidate for such a virus would be an agent that results in chronic infection and is transmissible by parenteral (and particularly sexual) routes. Clearly, WNV, dengue, and chikungunya failed to meet these expectations.

Model Viruses

Many studies of pathogen reduction have been performed using model viruses. There are a number of good reasons for this. Perhaps the most important is that there are no readily accessible infectivity assays for some of the key human transfusion-transmissible viruses, particularly HBV and HCV. Thus, closely related viruses have been used to provide guidance on the likely behavior of the human agents. For example, duck hepatitis virus (another hepadnavirus) has been used to simulate HBV, and bovine viral diarrhea virus, a pestivirus (a genus of the flaviviridae), has been used to simulate the related HCV.

In other circumstances, model viruses offer readily controlled experimental models and well-characterized starting materials. They can also be used to represent a much broader range of pathogens than those that are currently known to be transfusion transmitted. However, care has to be taken in interpreting all data from model viruses, as subtle structural differences can have an unexpectedly significant impact on susceptibility to viral inactivation procedures.

Bacteria

Bacterial contamination of blood components is not infrequent.[20] Bacteria may be introduced into blood from the donor's skin during the collection process (even in the face of scrupulous skin preparation methods), occasionally from the environment, and also as a result of low-level, asymptomatic bacteremia in the donor. Usually, the actual level of bacteria in the blood at the time of collection is too low to result in disease or sepsis in the recipient, although in some cases, actual infection might occur. More commonly, adverse effects on the recipient result from outgrowth of the contaminating bacteria during storage. This is of particular concern for platelets, which are stored at room temperature. Also, some psychrophilic bacteria can grow during long-term storage of red cells. Some data suggest that recipient sepsis or other adverse outcomes tend to be associated with higher levels of bacterial growth.[21]

Some improvement in bacterial safety has been achieved as a result of a complex of measures, such as by testing platelet units using automated bacterial culture, by improved skin preparation, and by diversion of the initial volume of collected blood.[22] It appears that residual sepsis is caused, in large part, by false-negative cultures as a result of the very low level of bacterial contamination at the time of sampling.[23] This provides an opportunity to estimate the actual levels of contamination in the collected product, generally thought to be significantly less than one viable bacterium per mL. Even in the absence of culture, it has been noted that initial levels of contamination are likely to be on this order, as outgrowth rarely, if ever, occurs in segments, even when heavy growth is eventually observed in the unit itself.

Parasites

A number of parasites are readily transmitted by transfusion, including those responsible for malaria, Chagas disease, and babesiosis. Current data suggest that actual levels of parasitemia among asymptomatic cases are relatively low.

For example, in most cases, at least in the United States, donors who have transmitted malaria have parasitemia levels below the level of detection of microscopy; that is, a few parasites per μL. Even so, this could imply as many as 10^6 parasites may be in a unit of blood: a substantial number, given estimates that 1 to 10 parasites may be enough to cause infection. Similarly, although in certain circumstances *Babesia* infection can result in incredible levels of parasitemia, the levels among asymptomatic individuals tend to be quite low.[24] This is also true for *T. cruzi*.

Prions and TSEs

Transmissible spongiform encephalopathies (TSEs) are a group of progressive, uniformly fatal neurologic diseases. It is widely accepted that the etiologic agent of TSEs, known as a prion, is a conformational variant of a naturally occurring protein, termed "PrP." It is thought that the pathologic form of this protein can recruit additional copies of the normal protein and act as a template for their conversion to the pathologic form, thus replicating or amplifying infectivity. The classic, prototypic human TSE is CJD, which occurs spontaneously at a frequency of about 1 case per million population. The disease may also be transmitted iatrogenically through shared use of neurosurgical instruments, certain tissue transplants, and pituitary-derived human growth hormone. A small minority of cases are associated with known gene mutations where the abnormal form of the prion arises spontaneously.

Animal-model studies have shown that there are high levels of TSE infectivity (perhaps 10^7 or more infectious doses per gram) in the brains of affected animals and that in some circumstances, low levels (perhaps around 10 infectious units per mL) may be found in the blood.[25] An important characteristic of TSE infectivity is that the agent is remarkably resistant to chemicals and processes normally used for sterilization or antisepsis.

The occurrence of classic CJD in an active blood donor has long been a matter of concern, although no study to date has identified any transmission by this route. Nevertheless, there are specific regulatory requirements designed to reduce the risk of donation by putatively affected individuals. However, it has recently become quite clear that vCJD, which results from infection with the prion of bovine spongiform encephalopathy, is transmissible by transfusion. There have been four cases in which the agent has been found in a recipient of blood that was collected from a donor who subsequently developed vCJD. Three of these cases resulted in fatal vCJD in the recipient.[1,26] Another case of apparent transmission of the agent by Factor VIII has also been described.[1] Transmission has been replicated in a sheep model.[27]

There are no published studies of the effects of current pathogen-reduction technologies on TSE infectivity, and it would not be anticipated that any of these approaches would have any degree of efficacy, even at the apparently modest levels that would be needed. However, some success has been achieved with affinity methods designed to remove prions from selected blood components.[28,29]

Cells

Blood components necessarily contain nucleated cells, even in circumstances in which measures have been taken to reduce the numbers of such cells. Leukocyte counts may be 10^9 to 10^{10} per unit, while standards for a leukocyte-reduced component require residual levels below 5×10^6 (US) or 1×10^6 (EU) per transfusible unit. It is widely recognized that viable leukocytes in transfused components may lead or contribute to adverse outcomes in the recipient, including alloimunization, transfusion-associated immune modulation, and graft-vs-host disease (GVHD). There is also increasing evidence that transfused cells may engraft and lead to long-term microchimerism, although it is not yet clear whether the condition has any pathogenic consequences. Certainly, GVDH is the most serious consequence of receipt of transfused leukocytes, and there are many circumstances in which components are irradiated to prevent this outcome. There is ample evidence that most pathogen-reduction technologies are able to prevent replication of leukocytes—indeed, in some cases, a very high level of DNA damage has been demonstrated. Animal-model studies have also shown that these methods can prevent the development of GVHD from infused cells.[30,31] In practice, some blood services have discontinued the use of product irradiation after implementation of pathogen reduction, even though there has been no definitive demonstration through clinical trials that the methods eliminate human GVHD.

Targets for Pathogen Reduction

Given the background outlined above, it may be possible to outline reasonable expectations for performance characteristics for a pathogen-reduction system. Perhaps the first question is whether pathogen reduction can meet the dream of a zero-risk blood supply. This author does not believe that such an expectation is realistic, at least in terms of what we know today. On one side of the issue, it is clear that there are a number of known viral agents that can reach high levels of infectivity (10^9 infectious units per mL or more) in the blood of asymptomatic individuals, and some of them (such as B19V) are quite resistant to current inactivation processes. Further, some, such as prions and selected viruses, appear to be completely resistant. It also seems unlikely that the potency of current methods of pathogen reduction can be increased significantly without compromising the therapeutic value of treated blood components. In addition, it is necessary to recognize that although the safety profiles of current methods are very high, there has not yet been enough experience to be certain that they will have no adverse effects at all.

At the other end of the spectrum, current data strongly suggest that addition of pathogen-reduction technologies, if used in addition to current blood safety measures, would have the capacity to essentially eliminate residual risk of infection from HBV, HCV, HIV, HTLV, WNV, *T. cruzi*, and bacterial contamination and syphilis infection. Moreover, it is very likely that risk from GVHD, malaria, and babesiosis would be materially reduced, if not eliminated. These outcomes could likely be accompanied by slight modification of some existing practices, such as the elimination of any need to consider single-donation testing by NAT and abandonment of bacterial culture and the use of irradiation to prevent GVHD. It might also be possible to argue for the elimination of NAT for HBV and testing for *T. cruzi* antibodies, HTLV antibodies, antibodies to hepatitis B core antigen, and syphilis. Further, arguments might be made for elimination or modification of some deferral policies, such as those for travel to areas at known but low risk of malarial infection. Some estimates of cost-effectiveness for existing technologies suggest that this level of outcome falls into the same range of marginal cost-effectiveness as other blood safety steps that have already been implemented.[32-34] While this range significantly exceeds that which is deemed acceptable for most medical interventions, it is a range that appears to be accepted for furtherance of blood safety.

There has been considerable speculation about the potential for eliminating other routine tests once pathogen reduction is routinely available. Ignoring the issues of regulatory barriers and of demonstrating the safety of this approach, an argument might be developed for relying only on a combination of NAT and pathogen reduction, as this approach would be expected to limit residual levels of virus to those that were within the demonstrated limits of effectiveness of inactivation procedures.

Although there is certainly something to be gained from the elimination of residual infectivity for known key pathogens, the ultimate promise of these technologies is as a proactive strategy to eliminate the risk of future outbreaks of as-yet-unknown transfusion-transmitted disease. For example, some question whether the transfusion transmissibility of WNV would ever have been discovered had pathogen reduction been in place. Published data for the efficacy of pathogen-reduction methods for platelets and plasma suggest that, at least in in-vitro studies, from 5.2 to 6.8 $\log_{10}$ of inactivation of WNV could be achieved. At the same time, the RNA levels in RNA-positive donors are generally less than 10^6 per mL. This suggests that the capacities of at least some inactivation processes are at a level where they might have the capacity to eliminate the maximal expected WNV infectivity from the volume of plasma in a red cell component but perhaps not in a full plasma unit. However, most donations do not have maximal levels of viremia, so a significant proportion of donations may indeed have been rendered noninfectious. It is not so clear that similar arguments could be applied to other arboviruses such as dengue and chikungunya; both of these viruses may be transmitted via a direct human-mosquito-human cycle and attain much higher levels of viremia in man (perhaps as many as 10^9 infectious doses per mL). Also, there is some evidence that other groups of viruses, particularly those that are nonenveloped, can show significant resistance to existing pathogen-reduction technologies, with only zero to 2-3 $\log_{10}$ of inactivation demonstrated.[1]

Although it is clear that it is not possible to predict the emergence of new infections, there is no doubt that there continues to be considerable concern about the possibility of an outbreak of a new disease with properties similar to HIV/AIDS. More specifically, the appearance of a chronic infection that has a very long, silent incubation period that could be missed through routine donor health history questions is worrisome. In retrospect, it is absolutely clear that an unexpectedly large number of individuals had been infected with HIV long before the first clinical cases were recognized. This included some 12,000 blood recipients in the United States alone. This is hardly surprising, given the fact that the time from infection to the appearance of AIDS was on the order of 10 years. Would pathogen-reduction technologies have prevented transfusion-related AIDS, had they been in place in 1970? It is certain that the methods used to inactivate viruses in pooled plasma products were completely successful in this regard, but this cannot be compared with the challenge offered by whole blood or labile components.

The profile of HIV markers in blood is now well known. After infection, there is a short eclipse phase with no detectable viral marker in the blood. A low level of infectivity may be seen just before the appearance of detectable RNA in the plasma. RNA levels increase steadily, with a doubling time of around 0.85 days. Levels peak at between 10^6 and 10^7/mL, then decline as antibodies are formed, followed by a lengthy steady state, with detectable RNA levels of 10^3 to 10^5 per mL. For the purposes of speculation, at least, a very conservative assumption might be that these levels reflect the maximal level of infectivity, but as pointed out above, this is probably a significant overestimate.

Published data show that pathogen-reduction techniques can remove greater than or equal to 6 logs of infectivity for HIV.[1] Because these represent the limit of measurement of the systems used, the maximal level is not known, although these levels do compare favorably with the RNA titers present in steady-state infection. It appears to be a reasonable assumption that pathogen-reduction technologies with currently recognized capacities would have a substantial impact on infectivity on at least a proportion, if not all, of these steady-state cases. Such an impact might be enough to eliminate infectivity from a red cell component and arguably might extend to a full unit of platelets or plasma. However, it is unclear whether the capacity of the process would extend to the levels of infectivity that might be present during the peak viremia period seen at the end of the ramp-up period. However, it must be recognized that, at any given time, this would represent only a very small proportion of infectious individuals.

Is it reasonable to anticipate that any future emergent infection with a lengthy incubation period would have a similar pattern of infectivity? It is really not possible to make a clear statement on this issue. What *is* known is that HBV likely attains and maintains higher infectivity levels than HIV, and this may also be true of some other persistent viruses.

Overall, then, it would be reasonable to anticipate that pathogen-reduction protocols as known today would reduce the incidence of transfusion transmission of an infection with properties comparable to those of HIV. Although it is not known with certainty that pathogen reduction would prevent the transmission of any and all infectious agents through transfusion, such a salutary outcome remains a possibility.

Definition of Efficacy of Pathogen Reduction

By necessity, the impact of pathogen reduction can only be inferred from the results of in-vitro and animal-model studies. Apart from the obvious ethical impossibility of performing studies on blood recipients, the frequency of residual infections is so low that it would not be possible to design a meaningful clinical or observational trial. Available laboratory data on inactivation of specific pathogens and model agents are posted on manufacturers' websites and/or incorporated into product information in Europe. Presumably, product claims for the United States will reflect the same data. This approach was used in the United States when pathogen reduction was introduced for plasma derivatives. However, it must be acknowledged that these data can serve only as a guide to reasonable expectations of efficacy such as those outlined above. Again, measures of infectivity based on tissue culture or animal models are not necessarily congruent with the levels observed in humans. Because the Food and Drug Administration licenses product claims on the basis of validated data produced by the manufacturer or during clinical trials, it appears unlikely that any formal claim of generic efficacy against unidentified emerging infections would be permitted in the United States. Such efficacy might nonetheless be inferred in some cases from data that are already available.

A further difficulty is that model systems may not permit measurement of the full range of inactivation that might be necessary to ensure elimination of all infectivity in a naturally occurring sample. Additional information and, more specifically, the actual kinetic curve of the inactivation process could help to interpret whether the actual level of inactivation would significantly exceed what can be measured. In some cases, such data are available in the scientific literature. As pointed out earlier, the actual infectious titer of blood components is also poorly characterized, as is the overall distribution of such titers. These facts make it difficult to develop a real-world estimate of the anticipated safety improvement that might be achievable through the use of any given pathogen-reduction technology. Further, the target inactivation efficacy for a desirable method is similarly difficult to define.

Summary and Conclusions

Information is sufficient to suggest that currently available pathogen-reduction technologies do have the potential to eliminate the threat of residual infectivity from major transfusion-transmissible pathogens, if used in conjunction with current tests. In addition, the use of such procedures would be expected to eliminate any risk of bacterial sepsis, even if current culture-based methods were discontinued, as has been done when the technology was implemented in parts of Europe. A case could also be made for eliminating irradiation and at least some serologic tests. Although it is likely that a significant but unpredictable proportion of infectious blood components could be rendered safe by pathogen reduction even in the absence of testing, it is not yet clear that total sterility could be ensured. The outlook concerning a hypothetical future infection is even more enigmatic, although in most cases it is likely that the impact of such an infection on blood safety would be materially reduced were pathogen reduction in place.

References

1. Stramer SL, Hollinger FB, Katz LM, et al. Emerging infectious disease agents and their potential threat to transfusion safety. Transfusion 2009;49(Suppl 2):1S-29S.
2. Barker LF, Shulman NR, Murray R, et al. Transmission of serum hepatitis. JAMA 1996;276:841-4.
3. Barker LF, Shulman NR, Murray R, et al. Transmission of serum hepatitis. JAMA 1970;211:1509-12.
4. Barker LF, Murray R. Acquisition of hepatitis-associated antigen. Clinical features in young adults. JAMA 1971;216:1970-6.

5. Kiyosawa K, Sodeyama T, Tanaka E, et al. Hepatitis C in hospital employees with needlestick injuries. Ann Intern Med 1991;115:367-9.
6. Henderson DK, Fahey BJ, Willy M, et al. Risk for occupational transmission of human immunodeficiency virus type 1 (HIV-1) associated with clinical exposures. A prospective evaluation. Ann Intern Med 1990;113:740-6.
7. Kleinman SH, Lelie N, Busch MP. Infectivity of human immunodeficiency virus-1, hepatitis C virus, and hepatitis B virus and risk of transmission by transfusion. Transfusion 2009;49:2454-89.
8. Kleinman SH, Busch MP. Assessing the impact of HBV NAT on window period reduction and residual risk. J Clin Virol 2006;36(Suppl 1):S23-9.
9. Busch MP, Glynn SA, Stramer SL, et al. A new strategy for estimating risks of transfusion-transmitted viral infections based on rates of detection of recently infected donors. Transfusion 2005;45:254-64.
10. Zou S, Stramer SL, Notari EP, et al. Current incidence and residual risk of hepatitis B infection among blood donors in the United States. Transfusion 2009;49:1609-20.
11. Stramer SL, Fang CT, Foster GA, et al. West Nile virus among blood donors in the United States, 2003 and 2004. N Engl J Med 2005;353:451-9.
12. Mohammed H, Linnen JM, Munoz-Jordan JL, et al. Dengue virus in blood donations, Puerto Rico, 2005. Transfusion 2008;48:1348-54.
13. Tambyah PA, Koay ES, Poon ML, et al. Dengue hemorrhagic fever transmitted by blood transfusion. N Engl J Med 2008;359:1526-7.
14. Chuang VW, Wong TY, Leung YH, et al. Review of dengue fever cases in Hong Kong during 1998 to 2005. Hong Kong Med J 2008;14:170-7.
15. Linnen JM, Broulik A, Collins C, et al. Detection of dengue virus RNA in blood donors from Honduras and Brazil with a prototype transcription-mediated amplification assay (abstract). Transfusion 2007;46(Suppl):38A.
16. Petersen LR, Stramer SL, Powers AM. Chikungunya virus: Possible impact on transfusion medicine. Transfus Med Rev 2010;24:15-21.
17. Liumbruno GM, Calteri D, Petropulacos K, et al. The chikungunya epidemic in Italy and its repercussion on the blood system. Blood Transfus 2008;6:199-210.
18. Rasongles P, Angelini-Tibert MF, Simon P, et al. Transfusion of platelet components prepared with photochemical pathogen inactivation treatment during a chikungunya virus epidemic in Ile de La Reunion. Transfusion 2009;49:1083-91.
19. Brown KE, Simmonds P. Parvoviruses and blood transfusion. Transfusion 2007;47:1745-50.
20. Eder AF, Kennedy JM, Dy B, et al for American Red Cross Regional Blood Centers. Bacterial screening of apheresis platelets and the residual risk of septic transfusion reactions: The American Red Cross experience (2004-2006). Transfusion 2007:47:1134-42.
21. Yomtovian RA, Palavecino EL, Dysktra AH, et al. Evolution of surveillance methods for detection of bacterial contamination of platelets in a university hospital, 1991 through 2004. Transfusion 2006;46:719-30.
22. Eder AF, Kennedy JM, Dy BA, et al. Limiting and detecting bacterial contamination of apheresis platelets: Inlet-line diversion and increased culture volume improve component safety. Transfusion 2009;49:1554-63.

23. Benjamin RJ, Wagner SJ. The residual risk of sepsis: Modeling the effect of concentration on bacterial detection in two-bottle culture systems and an estimation of false-negative culture rates. Transfusion 2007;47:1381-9.
24. Leiby DA. Babesiosis and blood transfusion: Flying under the radar. Vox Sang 2006;90:157-65.
25. Cervenakova L, Yakovleva O, McKenzie C, et al. Similar levels of infectivity in the blood of mice infected with human-derived vCJD and GSS strains of transmissible spongiform encephalopathy. Transfusion 2003;43:1687-94.
26. Hewitt PE, Llewelyn CA, Mackenzie J, Will RG. Creutzfeldt-Jakob disease and blood transfusion: Results of the UK Transfusion Medicine Epidemiological Review study. Vox Sang 2006;91:221-30.
27. Houston F, McCutcheon S, Goldmann W, et al. Prion diseases are efficiently transmitted by blood transfusion in sheep. Blood 2008;112:4739-45.
28. Sowemimo-Coker SO, Pesci S, Andrade F, et al. Pall leukotrap affinity prion-reduction filter removes exogenous infectious prions and endogenous infectivity from red cell concentrates. Vox Sang 2006;90:265-75.
29. Gregori L, Gurgel PV, Lathrop JT, et al. Reduction in infectivity of endogenous transmissible spongiform encephalopathies present in blood by adsorption to selective affinity resins. Lancet 2006;368:2226-30.
30. Grass JA, Wafa T, Reames A, et al. Prevention of transfusion-associated graft-versus-host disease by photochemical treatment. Blood 1999;93:3140-7.
31. Fast LD, DiLeone G, Cardarelli G, et al. Mirasol PRT treatment of donor white blood cells prevents the development of xenogeneic graft-versus-host disease in $Rag2^{-/-}$ gamma $c^{-/-}$ double knockout mice. Transfusion 2006;46: 1553-60.
32. Webert KE, Cserti CM, Hannon J, et al. Proceedings of a consensus conference: Pathogen inactivation—making decisions about new technologies. Transfus Med Rev 2008;22:1-34.
33. Moeremans K, Warie H, Annemans L. Assessment of the economic value of the INTERCEPT blood system in Belgium. Transfus Med 2006;16:17-30.
34. Postma MJ, van Hulst M, De Wolf JT, et al. Cost-effectiveness of pathogen inactivation for platelet transfusions in the Netherlands. Transfus Med 2005;15: 379-87.

In: AuBuchon JP, Prowse CV, eds.
Pathogen Inactivation: The Penultimate Paradigm Shift
Bethesda, MD: AABB Press, 2010

3

Toxicology Assessment of Pathogen-Inactivation Technologies: Amotosalen and Riboflavin Case Studies

RICHARD M. LEWIS, PHD, AND
JOY A. CAVAGNARO, PHD

ENSURING THE SAFETY OF A NOVEL TECHNOLOGY begins well before the initiation of human clinical trials. Extensive effort is applied to the evaluation of the possible toxicity of new drugs and devices in order to estimate the type, degree, and signs of adverse effects that might be observed in human use. Devices developed to manufacture pathogen-reduced blood products currently include two that add nucleic-acid-binding products, which are subsequently activated with ultraviolet (UV) light and (in one instance) re-

---

Richard M. Lewis, PhD, Chief Executive Officer, and Joy A. Cavagnaro, PhD, President, Access BIO, LC, Boyce, Virginia

R. Lewis and J. Cavagnaro have disclosed financial relationships with CaridianBCT and Cerus.

moved along with their by-products. Other technologies also have been developed. This review will focus on the amotosalen and riboflavin methods for platelet treatment because of their advanced development and use.

Throughout this volume, and this chapter in particular, the term "pathogen inactivation" (PI) is used to describe the removal of bacteria and viruses. Historically, the US Food and Drug Administration (FDA) has insisted on the term "pathogen reduction" to describe this process. In the regulatory sense, the removal of pathogens can never be ensured to be absolute, and "inactivation" implies total removal. Also, in experimental validation studies, if sufficiently high levels of a challenge agent are used, there still may be residual agents measured after inactivation. In order to be judged adequate, the amount of agent that is removed should exceed the anticipated real-life challenge by multiple orders of magnitude. Therefore, when the process removes a quantity of agents that is logs above what might be in the blood component, there is effectively complete removal. Moreover, the mechanism of action for amotosalen and for riboflavin and the respective treatment processes is a biochemical inactivation, because they use binding to nucleic acids to prohibit replication. Thus, the use of the term "inactivation" is consistent with the mechanism and the outcome of the methods.

Devices that add chemicals to (and remove them from) a biologic product offer both scientific and regulatory challenges for estimating their toxic potential. The evaluation is made more complex because these devices contain a drug and are used to manufacture a biologic drug. The process thus involves device regulation, small molecule drug regulation, and biologic blood product regulation. The toxicology evaluation must take into account the possible toxicity of the blood product after treatment, of the remaining inactivating agent itself, and the agent's residual components. In addition, devices that contact blood or body tissues must be tested for possible leachables and extractables and these evaluated for potential toxicity as well. Most of these toxicologic studies must be completed before clinical trials can begin. Thus, the majority of the toxicology evaluation is undertaken preclinically in studies appropriate to the planned clinical use of the blood product. The primary goal of most toxicity assessments is to provide some assurance of safety before the product enters clinical trials and, later, to evaluate possible long-term effects. Mechanistic toxicology studies may also be conducted to improve extrapolation. However, it is clinical trials and not the preclinical studies that provide the ultimate assessment of safety for approved products.

This discussion will address the toxicology programs of the Intercept (Cerus, Concord, CA), and Mirasol (CaridianBCT, Lakewood, CO) PI devices. Evaluation of the proper function of blood products after treatment for their efficacy and for product quality will be addressed in other chapters. In the cases of both the Intercept and Mirasol technologies, extensive testing for their ability to reduce the concentration of numerous infectious agents has been reviewed[1] and is also discussed elsewhere in this volume.

Regulation of Pathogen-Inactivation Technologies

The toxicity of the chemicals used in the PI technologies discussed here has been highlighted as one of a number of concerns regarding the implementation of these methods.[2,3] The transfusion community, PI developers, and regulatory authorities are encouraged to apply appropriate and established toxicology evaluations to ensure a high margin of safety for these methods.[2] As part of the marketing authorization, the FDA evaluates the toxicity potential of PI products. Although the PI methodologies rely basically on the use of specific devices, they are devices that are used to manufacture blood products. The FDA (Center for Biologics, Office of Blood Research and Review) evaluates the devices for the safety and efficacy of the product(s) that they manufacture in the same way as it evaluates apheresis instruments or blood bags and other devices used in the manufacturing of blood products.

The substances used in PI devices must, by nature, be very toxic to a broad range of pathogens but, at the same time, be highly selective in preventing damage to blood proteins and cells.[4] Amotosalen and riboflavin achieve these goals through their selective binding to nucleic acid and their activation in the presence of UV light.

Applicable Regulatory Guidance in Toxicity Testing

For the design of toxicology studies evaluating biotechnology-derived products, regulatory guidance is provided by the International

Conference on Harmonisation of Technical Requirements for Registration of Pharmaceuticals for Human Use (ICH). For biotechnology-derived pharmaceuticals (or biopharmaceuticals), the major guidance document is "Preclinical Safety Evaluation of Biotechnology-Derived Pharmaceuticals" (commonly referred to as "S6"), published in 1997.[5] A follow-up addendum is currently being developed. Although blood products are not specifically biotechnology-derived, this guidance is the most appropriate for designing preclinical safety programs for evaluating novel blood products. In S6 the recommended approach to preclinical safety evaluation is referred to as the "case-by-case" approach. This was largely based on the particular product's attributes with an understanding of the importance of defining relevant species for toxicity assessment in order to improve predictive value for humans. Throughout the document is the recognition of the probability of immunologically mediated effects on the toxicology testing and the possible relevance of species for evaluation and interpretation as well as determining if particular studies are necessary.[6] The application of S6 for evaluating novel plasma-derived products has been discussed.[7] ICH guidance for the timing of dosing in toxicology testing is provided by M3, "Nonclinical Safety Studies for the Conduct of Human Clinical Trials and Marketing Authorization for Pharmaceuticals."[8] Additional ICH guidance is provided for carcinogenicity testing (S1B), for genotoxicity (S2A, S2B, S2R1), for toxicokinetics (S3A), and pharmacokinetics (S3B).[9] Most toxicology testing is performed according to good laboratory practice (GLP) as defined in the US *Code of Federal Regulations* (CFR), 21 CFR, Part 58; however, for some studies, GLP may not be feasible, and an explanation can be given, allowing the data to be accepted and reviewed by the FDA.

As mentioned, because the blood products and the PI chemicals will be in contact with specific devices, regulatory agencies require a biocompatibility profile for the materials used in the device manufacturing. FDA has issued guidance on the development of such data and how International Organization for Standardization procedures should be used. At the same time, FDA recognizes that some devices are constructed of materials that have been previously used and characterized with a history of safe use. Therefore, not all tests suggested by the guidance are essential or needed for all devices.[10]

All toxicology testing may not be complete before the beginning of clinical trials. Certainly, sufficient testing to support the particular type and length of exposure as defined in a proposed clinical trial is performed before any human testing is begun. Sufficient preclinical animal testing will allow an estimate of the potential risk to the subjects and provide information to allow the subjects to give informed consent to participation in a trial. The toxicology data will allow the clinical investigators to exclude subjects who may be at greater risk, to be more aware of possible early indicators of toxicity, and to properly monitor studies for potential risks. Throughout the clinical development program, safety data are continually accumulated to contribute further to the risk estimate of the particular product for subsequent trials or ultimately for approval. The therapeutic index (TI) is the ratio between the drug dose that provides benefit and the dose that is toxic. The data to define the TI are developed in clinical trials. Before testing in humans, the margin of safety is estimated in animals. This margin is usually expressed as a multiple of the intended clinical dose, considering the animal dose at which toxic effects are observed.

Considerations in Preclinical Toxicology Study Design

The design of a toxicology program for a product will attempt to mimic the dosing parameters—for example, route, regimen, and delivery device—that are planned for the human clinical trials. The pharmacokinetics and dose volume of administration anticipated for humans will be considered in designing the selection and frequency of dose in the animal studies. The level of exposure is the primary consideration, and dosing in the animal studies should be sufficiently high to identify a toxicity signal and to define a toxic dose (or at least use a maximal feasible dose) and to observe a no-observed-adverse-effect level (NOAEL). The numbers of animals per sex per group should be sufficient to be able to recognize any possible gender-related effects. The definition of a relevant species is central to selection of species for testing. Unfortunately, it is often not possible to sufficiently power studies, especially when nonhuman primates are defined as the relevant species. In addition, when the material under evaluation is immunogenic in the animal species used, there are limitations in both study design as well as interpretation.

Because of the nature of the PI technologies and their inclusion of nucleic-acid-binding chemicals, particular attention has been paid to mutagenicity and, in the case of amotosalen (S-59), carcinogenicity evaluations.

An important component of determining toxicologic risk is the initial estimate of exposure. Animal models can be useful in this regard for estimating a range for the therapeutic dose to be tested for proof of concept in addition to determining toxicity. Exposure estimates will include consideration of route of administration and frequency of dosing to determine systemic concentrations. Of course, some knowledge of the intended clinical use will be needed as well as some pharmacokinetic predictions. Pharmacokinetic assessments provide important information for determining anticipated exposure to the product and, in the examples given here, to the toxic materials.

Analyses of the toxicologic risks associated with PI of platelets are used as examples in this chapter. Of these PI technologies, the most advanced in clinical trials are the Mirasol and Intercept systems. These methods add specific pathogen-inactivating compounds to the blood product. Thus the first toxicity determination is to estimate the possible exposure of subjects to these compounds in a worst-case scenario for the inactivation compound itself, for the reaction products generated by exposure to UV light, and for the treated blood product.

Intercept Technology

The Intercept device treats the blood component with amotosalen, a member of the chemical class of psoralens that, in the presence of light, photoalkylate the thymidine residues of DNA, resulting in inter- and intrachain crosslinks.[11] Psoralens in combination with UVA light have been used for many years in the therapy of melanoma in milligram quantities (0.6 mg/kg), taken orally before patient exposure to light.[12] Psoralen is a furocoumarin of which Americans are exposed to approximately 1.3 mg daily as part of their diets.[13] In the Intercept device this reaction takes place in the presence of platelets, and the excess amotosalen is adsorbed to an intradevice component. The toxicity of psoralen is seldom observed without simultaneous exposure to UV light.[11]

As mentioned above, because psoralens are similar to small molecule pharmaceuticals, a classical toxicology evaluation was used, including acute, subchronic, reproductive toxicity and other studies for the inactivating agent itself.[14] In order to develop a complete evaluation of the system, a number of the components were studied individually and together: the psoralen, amotosalen; amotosalen after exposure to UVA; amotosalen after exposure to UVA with adsorption; and finally, the blood component itself after all process steps had been applied to the platelet unit.

Genotoxicity and Carcinogenicity Assessments

Before in-vivo animal studies, an array of in-vitro tests of genotoxicity were performed using standard assay methods of evaluation in specific strains of bacteria (Ames testing with *Salmonella typhimurium* and *Escherichia coli*) and mammalian cells [mouse lymphocytes and Chinese hamster ovary (CHO) cells] as recommended in ICH S2B. Both amotosalen alone and amotosalen/UVA-treated platelets were evaluated for genotoxicty with and without the use of the adsorptive component of the device.[15,16] In addition, a number of studies were performed to try to increase the possible concentrations of photodegradation products. Because some drugs are more active after having been physiologically metabolized, tests are usually performed after incubation with preparations of rat liver microsomes. This can potentiate mutagenic effects. The genotoxicity assays were performed with and without metabolic activation of the compounds. One mutagenicity test out of six was positive. The dose used was 2000-fold higher than the anticipated clinical dose without metabolic activation, and 24,000-fold higher with activation.[15] Specific in-vivo tests for genotoxicity were performed in mice using the mouse micronucleus test and the unscheduled DNA synthesis test. Carcinogenicity was evaluated in the p53+/– transgenic mouse at three times/week dosing for 6 months. Because the genotoxicity testing was positive, it was appropriate to compare the dosage used in these studies with the estimated exposure to be used in the clinic. The carcinogenicity assessment was negative.

The anticipated clinical dose was 1 μg/kg amotosalen, 45 μg/kg free photoproducts, and 70 μg/kg bound photoproducts,[16,17] resulting in the calculated circulating amount of amotosalen of 1 ng/mL. As a result, the tested mutagenic concentration for these tests was more than 4×10^3 times and up to 7×10^6 times greater than that to be used in clinical practice.

The in-vitro effects were reported to be dose responsive, and no effects were observed in vivo. Generally when there is disagreement between in-vitro and in-vivo genotoxicity, the in-vivo results carry the most weight. In addition, the large safety margin for the in-vitro dose and the noted dose responsiveness at the higher doses suggest that the possible carcinogenic effects are negligible at the concentrations to be used clinically.[16] For amotosalen alone, the safety margins were >1000-fold for carcinogenicity, 100-fold for dermal toxicity, and 1000-fold for ocular toxicity in the phototoxicity studies. Thus, in spite of the known and observed mutagenicity and because of the lack of carcinogenicity and the high multiples for safety margins, the materials were judged to be safe at the anticipated concentrations to be used in the clinical trials.[16,17]

General Toxicity

Studies of amotosalen included subchronic 28-day (rat and dog) carcinogenicity and single-dose phototoxicity studies (albino rats). Amotosalen and radiolabeled amotosalen were used in pharmacokinetic, toxicokinetic, metabolism, excretion, and distribution studies. These studies were conducted with and without the use of the adsorptive device intended to remove excess amotosalen, and with and without UV exposure. These conditions were implemented in order to evaluate all possible concentrations and metabolites.[14,15] Treated platelets were not used in these studies.[15] The pharmacokinetic studies performed in mice and rats suggested a very rapid elimination half-life of 41 minutes as well as rapid metabolism. Similar studies were performed with 35% plasma (platelets are suspended in 35% plasma during amotosalen treatment). Because some of the amotosalen photoproducts bind to lipoproteins, in these studies using plasma, the elimination kinetics reflected rapid elimination of unbound materials and a longer time for elimination of bound materials.[14] Toxicokinetic studies were performed to determine if amotosalen induces degradative enzymes or if there is accumulation. In some studies after 3 months of dosing, there was some suggestion of enzyme induction in rats and some evidence of accumulation in dogs.

The exposure to the drug in these studies as measured by the maximum circulating concentration and the concentration over time was very high when compared to the exposure planned for initial human trials. Multiples of exposure ranged from 123 times to over 300 times the anticipated human exposure, yet the rate of reduction in concentration remained the same without observation of toxicity.

Extensive toxicity studies have been performed for amotosalen, as noted in Table 3-1.

No toxicity was noted in rat acute dosing studies performed with and without the adsorptive device. However, amotosalen alone was lethal at doses of 210 to 250 mg/kg. In acute studies in dogs, 40 mg/kg was not lethal but toxicity was observed. This toxicity was judged

Table 3-1. Toxicology Testing Performed for Amotosalen (S-59)*

Acute toxicity	Mutagenicity
Amotosalen	Amotosalen
Amotosalen illuminated	Amotosalen illuminated
With adsorptive device	Without adsorptive device
Without adsorptive device	Carcinogenicity
One-month	Amotosalen
Amotosalen	Amotosalen illuminated
Amotosalen illuminated	With adsorptive device
Without adsorptive device	Without adsorptive device
Three-month	Phototoxicity
Amotosalen illuminated	Amotosalen
With adsorptive device	Amotosalen illuminated
Without adsorptive device	With adsorptive device
Reproductive toxicity	Without adsorptive device
Amotosalen illuminated	
With adsorptive device	
Without adsorptive device	

*Various combinations of amotosalen with illumination and adsorption were performed. In addition to the studies listed, safety pharmacology studies of 25 mL/kg of the illuminated amotosalen mixture after adsorption using human platelets were conducted in monkeys for cardiovascular evaluation and in rats for renal and central nervous system studies.

to be insignificant based on the large safety margin (25,000-fold).[14,16,18]

In short-term, repeat-dose studies (subchronic) using daily dosing of various concentrations of amotosalen, illuminated and adsorbed, toxicity was observed for amotosalen at concentrations above 75 mg/kg/day in rats and 30 mg/kg/day in dogs. Monkey studies with human platelets were stopped early, around 6 weeks, because of immunologic reactions to the human platelets and plasma, an outcome that was not unexpected. The ability to alter the antigenic conformation of the platelets and the suspending 35% plasma by amotosalen illumination and adsorption was further assessed in initial clinical trials.[19]

Studies similar to those described for platelets also have been performed for plasma PI using the amotosalen technology.[15]

Reproductive toxicology studies for amotosalen included assessments in male and female rats, teratology evaluations in rats and rabbits, and peri/postnatal evaluations in rats.

Because of the potential use of Intercept to treat platelets intended for transfusion in neonates, a toxicology study was performed to evaluate possible effects of amotosalen in a model animal population. Neonatal rats received daily infusions from 1 µg/kg/day up to 457 µg/kg/day from postnatal day 4 to postnatal day 31. Animals were evaluated for effects on many toxicologic parameters without noted toxicity.[20]

The amotosalen studies for the Intercept technology were extensive and investigated many parameters of possible exposure. The studies were conducted over a wide range of concentrations and preparation methods. The predominant toxicity signal was noted at concentrations over 25,000-fold higher than that used for clinical trials, providing a wide safety margin.

Mirasol Technology

Riboflavin (vitamin B2) is a naturally occurring compound that, in its coenzyme form, is a human physiologic component of oxidation-reduction reactions and participates in energy production. Riboflavin is listed by the FDA as a GRAS substance, meaning "generally recognized as safe" as a food additive[21] and is an essential nutrient with a recommended daily (oral) allowance of 0.4 to 1.6

mg/day, depending on age and gender.[22] Although ordinarily ingested, riboflavin is included during parenteral nutrition at recommended levels of 1.8 to 5.4 mg/day, depending on age,[23] up to 11.6 mg/day.[24] Toxicity levels reported in the literature are >10 mg/kg taken orally, 5 mg/kg with subcutaneous injection, and 560 μg/kg after intraperitoneal injection.[25] It should be noted that absorption through the oral route is limiting. Because riboflavin is an essential nutrient, there is sufficient literature on the necessary minimal levels of intake for good health but limited literature on toxic levels. As a water-soluble vitamin, riboflavin does not accumulate physiologically, and when excess amounts are administered, increased urinary excretion of the compound occurs.[26] In fact, it has been reported that urinary excretion accounts for up to one-half of the overall removal of riboflavin from plasma.[24] Further, the longstanding use of riboflavin with phototherapy for neonatal jaundice has proven safe.[27] Importantly for PI use, riboflavin has been demonstrated to increase the light-sensitivity of nucleic acid and diminish its ability for repair.[28] The toxicity profile of riboflavin was comprehensively reviewed in the context of the Mirasol toxicology program.[29]

Pharmacokinetic studies using Mirasol-treated plasma containing radiolabeled riboflavin suggest a short half-life of 52 hours. More than half of the labeled material was excreted in the urine within 12 hours.[29]

Genotoxicity Assessment

The battery of tests for genotoxicity in riboflavin is very similar to that described for psoralen, including Ames tests with and without activation, mammalian cells, and CHO cells, as recommended in ICH S2B. In addition, Ames testing was performed with lumichrome, the primary photodegradation product of riboflavin.

Unlike amotosalen, no tests were positive for riboflavin genotoxicity, and carcinogenicity testing was not performed. The completely negative genotoxicity testing, in itself, is not reason to omit carcinogenicity testing but contributes to the rationale for excluding such studies. That rationale was based on the further evaluation of photodegradation products, the absence of any indication of tumorigenic potential in the toxicity tests, the chemical nature of the molecule, and the long human experience in the evaluation and testing of riboflavin.[29]

General and Reproductive/Developmental Toxicity

In spite of the confidence in the safety of riboflavin administered orally and intravenously as a nutrient, the possible toxic effects after illumination in the Mirasol device and the effects of its photoreaction products were evaluated in an extensive toxicology program (Table 3-2).

The major toxicity concerns for riboflavin are the effects of the breakdown products after UV light, exposure in the presence of

Table 3-2. Toxicology Testing Performed for Mirasol*

Acute
Rat
Riboflavin, illuminated
Treated platelets—2 injections†
Treated and γ-irradiated platelets—1 injection
Treated and γ-irradiated platelets—2 injections
Treated and γ-irradiated platelets—3 injections
Dog
Treated platelets—2 injections†
Treated and γ-irradiated platelets—1 injection
Treated and γ-irradiated platelets—2 injections
Treated and γ-irradiated platelets—3 injections
Subchronic
Dog
Riboflavin solution, illuminated—1 injection
Riboflavin solution, illuminated—3 injections
Reproductive toxicity
Rats
Treated plasma

*Various combinations of riboflavin with illumination and adsorption were performed.

†When multiple injections were given for the acute studies, they were given 2 hours apart.

blood components, and the toxicity of the blood products themselves after treatment by the chemicals and device.

Two acute toxicity studies in rats and dogs used platelets from the particular species treated using the Mirasol technology and either irradiation or no irradiation. In addition, an acute study was performed without the inclusion of platelets in order to increase the levels of riboflavin and its photoproducts. Dogs were used for the subchronic study of Mirasol-treated platelets, which used 13 weeks of daily dosing with a 4-week recovery period. No positive findings were reported for any group in any of these studies.[29]

Reproductive toxicity was evaluated in rats using rat plasma treated with the Mirasol system. No effects were observed for fetal weight, fetus viability, litter size, and other standard measures. It is interesting to note that treated dams showed significant weight gain related to food consumption.

In the data reported for all of these animal studies, there was no indication of toxicity of the Mirasol process at those doses tested. The preclinical toxicity program for Mirasol was somewhat more limited than that reported for amotosalen because of the nature of the product. The doses tested encompassed a wide range of concentrations that would provide a reasonable safety margin for further human trials.

Conclusion

Both PI examples described underwent extensive toxicology evaluations. The mode of action of the compounds is very similar in that they bind nucleic acids and become covalently attached through UVA light activation. Riboflavin has been studied extensively as a nutritional requirement.[22,30] The toxicity of riboflavin in the context of light exposure of treated individuals has also been studied,[27] and toxicity testing has been limited only by its solubility.[25] Although some psoralens (eg, 8-methoxypsoralen) have been used with photoactivation for therapy, their potential for increasing carcinogenicity has also been recognized.[11,31] In the case of amotosalen and riboflavin technologies, the safety margins, which are multiples of toxicity concentrations, are very high depending on the measure, ranging in orders of magnitude from $>10^2$ to $>10^5$. Thus, the safety margins that were defined preclinically for Intercept and Mirasol were judged sufficient to support clinical trials. In addition, there was no apparent toxicity in animal testing to suggest immediate concern. One of the primary aims of toxicology testing is to estimate safety margins to better inform clinical researchers. It is on this base of information that clinical testing is justified and the safety profile is further expanded. Occasionally, novel toxicities are identified during clinical testing, and the need arises to further investigate their nature in animal studies. Assessment of safety is an iterative process.

Preclinical toxicology testing is limited in defining the ultimate safety of a product. Small numbers of animals in cross-species testing are used to attempt to predict responses in humans. Although the system has been useful for small molecule pharmaceuticals, biologic products are more difficult to evaluate, often because of unique species specificity and/or immunogenicity when testing human-derived molecules in animals.

A toxicology program will enable clinical trials with an acceptable margin of safety. Based on the differences in species; the number of animals tested; the nature of the toxicity, including reversibility; and the ability to monitor for the specific toxicity in humans, an additional safety factor may be added (eg, 10×) to provide even greater reassurance of safety.

Thus, the preclinical safety evaluation does not provide assurance of safety of a marketed product but forms the basis of a much larger database that is formed primarily of clinical research and postmarketing surveillance to continually improve understanding of product safety.

References

1. Wu YY, Snyder EL. Safety of the blood supply: Role of pathogen reduction. Blood Rev 2003;17:111-22.
2. Klein HG, Anderson D, Bernardi MJ, et al. Pathogen inactivation: Making decisions about new technologies. Report of a consensus conference. Transfusion 2007;47:2338-47.
3. Webert KE, Cserti CM, Hannon J, et al. Proceedings of a consensus conference: Pathogen inactivation—making decisions about new technologies. Transfus Med Rev 2008;22:1-34.
4. Chapman J. Toxicology considerations relating to the pathogen inactivation of blood products: Potential for impact on recipients. Presented at the 33rd

meeting of the US Public Health Service Advisory Committee on Blood Safety and Availability, Washington, DC, January 9, 2008 (transcript). Washington, DC: Department of Health and Human Services, 2008. [Available at http://www.hhs.gov/ophs/bloodsafety/pastmeetings/transcripts/acbsa080109.pdf (accessed April 22, 2010).]

5. International Conference on Harmonisation of Technical Requirements for Registration of Pharmaceuticals for Human Use. ICH harmonized tripartite guideline: Preclinical safety evaluation of biotechnology-derived pharmaceuticals; S6. Step 4 version. CPMP/ICH/302/95. (July 16, 1997) Geneva: ICH, 1997. [Available at http://www.ich.org/LOB/media/MEDIA503.pdf (accessed April 21, 2010).]
6. Cavagnaro J. Preclinical safety evaluation of biotechnology-derived pharmaceuticals. Nat Rev Drug Discov 2003;1:469-75.
7. Lewis RM, Cavagnaro J. The application of ICH S6 to the preclinical safety evaluation of plasma derivative therapeutic products. Annapolis, MD: Plasma Protein Therapeutics Association, 2009. [Available on the PPTA Web site (Issues>US>regulatory>manufacturing) at http://www.pptaglobal.org/UserFiles/file/RPSC09053a_Application%20of%20S6%20to%20Plasma-Derivatives%20FINAL_August%202009.pdf (accessed April 22, 2010).]
8. ICH Topic M3(R2). Non-clinical safety studies for the conduct of human clinical trials and marketing authorization for pharmaceuticals. CPMP/ICH/286/95. (July 2008) London: European Medicines Agency, 2008. [Available at http://www.ema.europa.eu/pdfs/human/ich/028695endraft.pdf (accessed April 22, 2010).]
9. International Conference on Harmonisation of Technical Requirements for Registration of Pharmaceuticals for Human Use. Safety guidelines. New codification as per November 2005. Geneva: ICH, 2010. [Available at http://www.ich.org/cache/compo/502-272-1.html (accessed April 22, 2010).]
10. Food and Drug Administration. Use of international standard ISO-10993, "Biological evaluation of medical devices part 1: Evaluation and testing." (Replaces #G87-1 #8294) (blue book memo). (May 1, 1995) Silver Spring, MD: CDRH Office of Device Evaluation, 1995. [Available at http://www.fda.gov/MedicalDevices/DeviceRegulationandGuidance/GuidanceDocuments/ucm080735.htm (accessed April 22, 2010).]
11. Wollowitz S. Fundamentals of the psoralen-based Helinx technology for inactivation of infectious pathogens and leukocytes in platelets and plasma. Semin Hematol 2001;38(Suppl):4-11.
12. Dover JS, Stern RS. Psoralens new formulation! Better formulation? Arch Dermatol 1986;122:763-5.
13. Wagstaff DJ. Dietary exposure to furocoumarins. Regul Toxicol Pharmacol 1991;14:261-72.
14. Ciaravino V, McCullough T, Dayan AD. Pharmacokineitic and toxicology assessment of Intercept (S-59 and UVA treated) platelets. Hum Exp Toxicol 2001;20:533-50.
15. Ciaravino V, McCullough T, Cimino G, Sullivan T. Preclinical safety profile of plasma prepared using the Intercept blood system. Vox Sang 2003;85:171-82.

16. Tice R, Gatehouse D, Kirkland D, Speit G. The pathogen reduction treatment of platelets with S-59 HCl (amotosalen) plus ultraviolet A light: Genotoxicity profile and hazard assessment. Mutat Res 2007;630:50-68.
17. Cerus Corporation. S-59 Photochemical treatment of platelet concentrates (FDA briefing package). Presented at the FDA Blood Products Advisory Committee meeting, Bethesda, MD, November 16-17, 2009.
18. Dayan AD. The science of safety: Toxicological review of amotosalen HCl. Transfus Med Hemother 2004;31(Suppl 1):17-23.
19. Lin L, Conlan MG, Tessman J, et al. Amotosalen interactions with platelet and plasma components: Absence of neoantigen formation after photochemical treatment. Transfusion 2005;45:1610-20.
20. Ciaravino V, Hanover J, Lin L, et al. Assessment of safety in neonates for transfusion of platelets and plasma prepared with amotosalen photochemical pathogen inactivation treatment by a 1-month intravenous toxicity study in neonatal rats. Transfusion 2009;49:985-94.
21. Food and Drug Administration. Database of Select Committee on GRAS Substances (SCOGS) Reviews: Riboflavin. Rockville, MD: FDA, 1979. [Available at http://www.accessdata.fda.gov/scripts/fcn/fcnDetailNavigation.cfm?rpt=scogsListing&id=272 (accessed April 22, 2010).]
22. Institute of Medicine. Dietary reference intakes for thiamin, riboflavin, niacin, vitamin B6, folate, vitamin B12, pantothenic acid, biotin, and choline. Washington, DC: National Academies Press, 2000.
23. Marinier E, Gorski AM, de Courcy GP, et al. Blood levels of water-soluble vitamins in pediatric patients on total parenteral nutrition using a multiple vitamin preparation. JPEN J Parenter Enteral Nutr 1989;13:176-84.
24. Zempleni J, Galloway J, McCormick D. Pharmacokinetics of orally and intravenously administered riboflavin in healthy humans. Am J Clin Nutr 1996; 63:54-66.
25. Unna K, Geslin J. Studies on the toxicity and pharmacology of riboflavin. J Pharmacol Exp Ther 1942;76:75-80.
26. McCormick DB. Two interconnected B vitamins: Riboflavin and pyridoxine. Physiol Rev 1989;69:1170-98.
27. Olsen JH, Hertz H, Kjaer SK, et al. Childhood leukemia following phototherapy for neonatal hyperbilirubinemia. Cancer Causes Control 1996;7:411-14.
28. Kumar V, Lockerbie O, Keil SD, et al. Riboflavin and UV-light based pathogen reduction: Extent and consequences of DNA damage at the molecular level. Photochem Photobiol 2004;80:15-21.
29. Reddy H, Dayan AD, Cavagnaro J, et al. Toxicity testing of a novel riboflavin-based technology for pathogen reduction and white blood cell inactivation. Transfus Med Rev 2008;22:133-53.
30. Powers H. Riboflavin (vitamin B-2) and health. Am J Clin Nutr 2003;77: 1352-60.
31. Honig B, Morison WL, Karp D. Photochemotherapy beyond psoriasis. J Am Acad Dermatol 1994;31:775-90.

In: AuBuchon JP, Prowse CV, eds.
Pathogen Inactivation: The Penultimate Paradigm Shift
Bethesda, MD: AABB Press, 2010

4

Pathogen Inactivation of Red Cell Components

JOSE A. CANCELAS, MD, PHD

THREE CIRCUMSTANCES, EACH DESCRIBED AGAIN elsewhere in this text, have favored the persistence of infection transmissibility as a major problem in cell component therapies in the United States and Europe: 1) the occurrence of infections during the window period of detection, 2) the possibility of infection transmission by components containing a low pathogen copy number, and 3) the emergence of pathogens for which licensed tests are not

---

Jose A. Cancelas, MD, PhD, Division Director, Research, Hoxworth Blood Center and Director, Flow Cytometry Core Facility, Division of Experimental Hematology and Cell Biology, Cincinnati Children's Hospital Medical Center, University of Cincinnati Academic Health Center, Cincinnati, Ohio

The author has disclosed no conflicts of interest.

available. These pathogens include viruses—such as parvovirus B19 and hepatitis A, flaviviruses [other than West Nile virus (WNV)], herpesvirus-8 (HHV-8), hepatitis E, hepatitis G, SEN, TT, severe acute respiratory syndrome coronavirus, avian or swine influenza, Colorado tick fever, and tick-borne encephalitis—as well as a growing group of bacteria (eg, *Yersinia enterocolitica*) and an emergent group of protozoa infections, including *Trypanosoma cruzi* (for which testing is now performed) and other pathogens for which there are no tests, such as *Babesia* sp., *Anaplasma phagocytophilum*, and *Rickettsia rickettsii*.

These factors may support the use of pathogen inactivation (PI) technologies. In addition, treatment with ionizing radiation to prevent transfusion-associated graft-vs-host disease (TA-GVHD)[1] is associated with a reduction in cell component shelf life and with accelerated release of potassium into the extracellular medium,[2] which results in the need for two blood component inventories in hospitals.[3] PI inactivates leukocytes and can substitute for irradiation.

Finally, transfusion-related alloimmunization (TR-AI) and immunomodulation (TRIM) involve alloimmunization and immunosuppression, respectively, associated with transfusion. These have been associated with leukocyte antigens (especially HLA) and leukocyte-derived compounds (including Fas ligand, tumor necrosis factor, and soluble HLA substances). The implementation of universal leukocyte reduction resulted in a significant decrease in alloimmunization and immunosuppression associated with transfusion.[4] Nonetheless, some leukocytes persist and are believed to remain a source of alloimmunization and immunosuppression after transfusion.[5-8] Recent biologic data have suggested that the use of PI may reduce TR-AI.[9]

Pathogen Inactivation—Considerations for Red Cells

PI has been proposed as a complement, or even a possible alternative, to the screening methods currently employed. The use of PI aims to reduce or eliminate viable pathogens and inactivate leukocytes in donated blood.[10,11]

Despite the refrigeration of red cells during storage, red cell components have been shown to retain the potential for viral and prion transmission and to allow survival of bacterial and parasitic pathogens, including bacteria as diverse as *Y. enterocolitica,*[12-13] *Streptococcus pneumoniae,*[14] and exotic parasitic infections such as *Loa loa.*[15] Development of PI methods for red cell components is at an earlier stage than that for plasma and platelets, which are considered elsewhere in this text.

The significant cost and the logistical requirements associated with the use of PI all favor the idea of validating PI methods that can be applied to whole blood before component production. These methods would allow single-step PI, facilitate the process and logistics of PI implementation, and significantly reduce the cost of the procedure compared with alternative, component-specific PI methods. Effective methods for PI of whole blood and red cell components can be divided into two categories: physical PI and chemical PI.

Physical Methods for Red Cells

Physical reduction methods physically remove pathogenic particles and the blood cells that contain those particles. These methods include leukocyte reduction, plasma reduction, extensive washing, and controlled freezing/thawing.

Leukocyte Reduction

The widespread use of leukocyte-reduction filters that are able to reduce residual leukocytes by >4 $\log_{10}$ has significantly reduced the frequency of leukocyte-transmitted viral diseases. These filters have resulted in a significant reduction in the transmissibility of cytomegalovirus (CMV), a virus that has been shown to be exclusively transmitted by leukocytes,[16] allowing many communities to develop "CMV-reduced-risk" blood inventories without testing for seronegativity, although these are still controversial.[17,18] Leukocyte reduction has probably had an impact on the transmissibility of human T-cell lymphotropic viruses (HTLV),[19,20] which are believed to be transmitted only by leukocytes, although recent data have shown that some infectivity of these viruses, as assessed by microbiologic culture, persists despite leukocyte reduction.[21,22] Generally, leukocyte reduction is associated with approximately 10% loss of the component[23,24] and is usually the first phase among the other physical and chemical methods for PI because of the extent of its pathogen-removal effect.

Prion Filtration of Red Cells

Combining leukocyte reduction with more refined filtration technologies based on affinity chromatography has been shown to be the only feasible method of PI for red cells that prevents the transmission of prion-related disease (using spiked blood models of prion disease).

Leukocyte-reduction filters can remove ~40% of endogenous prions from blood.[25] A prion filter based on the use of the resin L13A[25,26] has been shown to deplete around 4 $\log_{10}$ infectivity in human blood spiked with 263K scrapie-infected hamster brain homogenate, a commonly used model to test prion infectivity. At least 1.2 $\log_{10}$ of infectivity was removed from the blood of scrapie-infected hamsters. Red cell storage parameters have been evaluated for leukocyte-reduced red cells filtered with the P-Capt (MacoPharma, Tourcoing, France) prion filter and stored with either plasma-citrate-phosphate-dextrose or saline-adenine-glucose-mannitol until outdate.[27] No effects on complement or coagulation factor systems were observed, and no platelet activation was identified. The red cells filtered through the P-Capt prion filter also maintained acceptable biochemical parameters and in-vivo 24-hour radiolabeled red cell recoveries; there was an apparent absence of neoantigen formation after autologous infusion of an individual treated red cell unit.[28,29] Three other prion-absorbent filters have been recently tested and shown to have significant prion-reduction capability,[30] and two of them have recently been approved for use in Europe.

Chemical Methods for Red Cells

Because of the limited efficacy of physical procedures, chemically based PI technologies have been developed. These require permeation of chemicals or byproducts into blood cells and/or pathogens, without damaging the blood cell function or creating neoantigens, and the effective inactivation of extracellular and intracellular pathogens.

Photochemical PI of whole blood or red cell concentrates has faced major drawbacks. There are three primary difficulties: 1) the ability of hemoglobin to absorb or scatter light; 2) the need for "significant" retention of storage stability, including in-vivo recovery and survival; and 3) the need for the process to avoid neoantigen formation. Because of these challenges, no PI method for red cells has yet been shown to have completely satisfactory results in clinical trials.

Two types of chemical PI methods have been used, those that use chemicals that require photoactivation or those that do not.

Chemicals That Do Not Require Photoactivation

Some chemicals have been developed with the aim of solving the technical problems associated with the use of photoactivated chemicals and light exposure. These chemicals directly cross-link nucleic acids, and hence impair their transcription and replication.

Inactine PEN110

The ethyleneimine oligomers are a group of chemicals for PI that includes Inactine or PEN110 (formerly, of Vitex, Watertown, MA).[31-44] PEN110 (see Fig 4-1) is a low-molecular-weight, highly water-soluble cation, that diffuses rapidly across the cell membrane. It then selectively binds to nucleic acid guanidine bases (position N-7), and undergoes activation after binding to negatively charged phosphate groups at a neutral pH. This results in alkylation of the imidazole ring structure of guanidine, and the breakage of the nucleic acid strand with disruption of transcription and replication. After treatment, excess PEN110 is removed by washing before storage. The method has been shown to be highly effective in viral reduction. Specifically, latent CMV and WNV are highly susceptible to this process. A Phase I clinical trial of 28-day stored, PEN110-treated red cells has shown red cell in-vivo recovery similar to controls, albeit with shortened survivals.[31,33,34,40] PEN110 treatment, although not severely harmful to red cells, did cause antibody formation

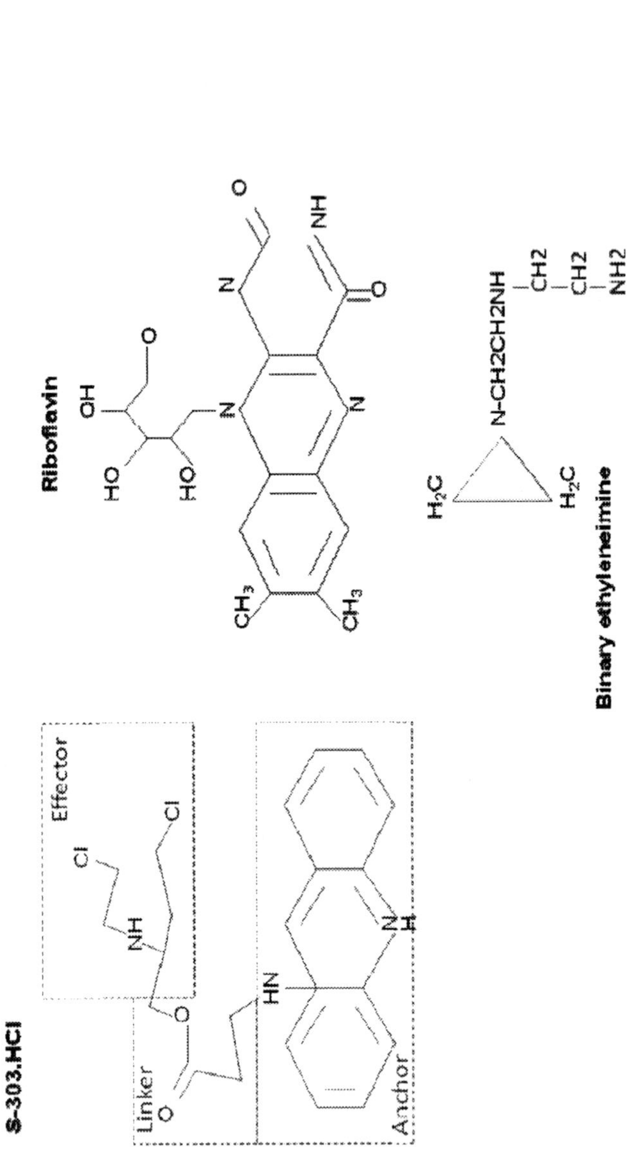

Figure 4-1. Chemical structure of the three molecules used in red cell pathogen reduction in clinical trials (PEN110 is an ethylene-imine oligomer).

against treated red cells in two sickle cell anemia patients following repeated transfusions. There were no recognized clinical consequences of the antibody formation, and the nature of the immune responses and the specificities of the antibodies formed in the PEN110 trials have not been reported.

The company that was developing this approach has abandoned the project, and no further studies have been conducted in the past 5 years, making further development of the technology unlikely. A summary of PEN110 activity and red cell in-vivo recovery and survival is included in Tables 4-1 and 4-2.

S-303

A more promising candidate is S-303 (Helinx; see Fig 4-1), a positively charged, alkylating agent derived from quinacrine mustard with a planar structure that has been developed by Cerus Corporation (Concord, CA).[45,48,49] S-303 contains an intercalator group that inserts into the helical region of the nucleic acid, and an effector group that allows covalent modification of nucleic acid with a central frangible bond, enabling degradation of the compound. Activation and cross-linking occurs on transfer from a low-pH environment to the neutral pH of blood. The process is completely light independent. The primary byproduct of S-303 degradation is S-300, which is rapidly metabolized and excreted, leaving no residual parent compound detectable by mass spectroscopy. Glutathione (GSH), a naturally occurring substance present in most cells of the body at millimolar concentrations, is used as an extracellular quencher of the reaction to inhibit surface modification of red cells. In the original protocol, residual S-303 degradation products were adsorbed and removed by a compound adsorption device (CAD).

S-303 has demonstrated inactivation of a wide range of viruses, bacteria, and protozoa.[50] Tests for teratogenicity, carcinogenicity, and mutagenicity, both in vitro and in animal models, were universally negative. In-vitro analysis of red cell metabolic status [adenosine 5′-triphosphate (ATP), 2,3-diphosphoglycerate, glucose consumption, lactate production, potassium leakage, and hemolysis] were comparable to control red cells. Despite S-303 binding to the red cell membrane and intracellular proteins, red cell in-vivo recovery and survival[45] was comparable to control red cells in three dif-

Table 4-1. Comparison of Methods Used for PI in Clinical Trials

Comparable Feature	S-303*	Inactine/PEN110†	Mirasol‡
Active compound	Frangible anchor linker with an acridine-based effector (FRALE)	Ethyleneimine oligomers with cationic tail conferring DNA binding	Riboflavin and visible (blue) or ultraviolet light
Photoactivation	No	No	Yes
Target	Nucleic acids	Nucleic acids	Nucleic acids
Bystander targets	Proteins and potentially lipids	Proteins	Possibly proteins and lipids
Toxicity	Very low after frangible anchor breaks off	Very low	Very low
Removal of active compounds	CAD or washing step with saline	Washing step with saline	No
Bacteria reduction	3 to >6 $\log_{10}$	3 to >6 $\log_{10}$	3 to >6 $\log_{10}$
Lipid-enveloped virus reduction	4 to >6 $\log_{10}$	4 to >6 $\log_{10}$	4 to >6 $\log_{10}$
Nonenveloped virus reduction	>4 $\log_{10}$	>4 $\log_{10}$	Variable
WBC inactivation	High	High	High
Effect on alloimmunization	Not investigated	Not investigated	Reduction in vitro and in animal models
Prion inactivation	Depletion depends on washing step (in protocols including washing)	Depletion dependent on extent of washing	Depletion depends on washing step (in protocols including washing)

Complexity of method	Addition of reagent plus neutralizing glutathione and use of CAD or washing	Addition of reagent, dilution, and washing step	Addition of reagent and illumination
Antibody formation (in vivo)	• No antibody development in Phase Ia, Ib, and Ic studies, which include serial transfusion of healthy subjects, and in acute transfusion Phase III study. • Development of antibodies in two serially-transfused hemoglobinopathy patients (out of 17 patients serially transfused and 50 enrolled)	After Phase I and II clinical studies; Phase III studies abandoned because of development of antibodies against PEN110-treated red cells in two of 70 enrolled patients	Untested
Stage of process development (end of 2009)	• Changes in GSH use and concentration (10-fold increase) • Changes in storage additive solution (2nd protocol) • Addition of washing step (3rd protocol)	Discontinued development	• Development of whole blood PI in progress • Determination of adequate light intensity to preserve red cell viability and function while maintaining PI and WBC inactivation

*Cerus Corp, Concord, CA.
†Vitex, Watertown, MA.
‡CaridianBCT, Lakewood, CO.
PI = pathogen inactivation; CAD = compound adsorption device; WBC = white (blood) cell; GSH = glutathione.

Table 4-2. Comparison of Red Cell Viability and Metabolic Parameters between S-303 and PEN110 Methods

Method	Stored Red Cell 24-hour ^{51}Cr Recovery (vs control; %)	Survival T50 (vs control; days)	Hemolysis (%)	ATP (vs control: umoles/g Hb)
S-303 (35-day storage)[45-47]	1st protocol*: 78.7 - 84.4 (82.6 - 84.5) 2nd protocol†: 79.8 (84.4) 3rd protocol†: 88 (90)	1st protocol*: 38.4 (38.6) 2nd protocol†: 43.7 (54.1) 3rd protocol†: 33 (40)‡	<1	2nd protocol†: 2.7 (3.1)
PEN110[33]	85 (86) (28-day storage)	31.9 (32.9) (28-day storage)	0.70 (0.23)	1.79 (2.89) (42-day storage)

*Range of averages of three Phase I studies, including 42 subjects (21 test and 21 control) with single exposure, 28 subjects (12 test and 16 control) with multiple exposure, and 29 subjects in a crossover trial.
†Average of a trial including 27 subjects in a crossover design.
‡Interim analysis of test and control red cell survival.
T50 = lapse of time in which 50% of the circulating red cells disappear; ATP = adenosine triphosphate.

ferent Phase I clinical trials where serial infusion of S-303-treated red cells was performed. In these normal volunteers, no formation of S-303 antibodies was noticed. Two Phase III clinical trials have been published. The first randomized study was applied to acute transfusion in patients undergoing cardiac surgery, of which 148 patients were evaluable. No differences were observed in the efficacy endpoint of treatment-related morbidity or mortality or in their transfusion needs. The safety profile was adequate, as no relevant differences in adverse events were noticed, and there was identical frequency of neoantibody formation (two of 74 patients) in the group who received S-303 red cells and the control group.[49] The second randomized Phase III clinical trial, in patients receiving chronic transfusion for thalassemia and sickle cell disease, was suspended following development of antibodies against S-303-treated red cells in two of 17 multiply transfused patients.[49] The antibodies did not induce hemolysis in vivo or in vitro in macrophage monolayer assays.[51] Further research demonstrated that the specific protocol used to treat red cells with S-303 induced alloimmunization in sensitive animal models.[48]

Modifications of the original S-303 protocol, by increasing the concentration of GSH and changing the pH of the treatment additive solution, allow PI in red cells and whole blood, with an excellent PI profile. Furthermore, this modified system does not induce red cell alloimmunization in sensitive animal models. Excellent red cell metabolic status is maintained in vitro.[48] In-vivo studies on modified S-303 PI technology are ongoing. Preliminary data suggest that the life span of red cells treated with S-303 may be modestly shortened.[46] A summary of S-303 activity and red cell in-vivo recovery and survival are included in Tables 4-1 and 4-2. Changes in the storage additive solution for red cells treated with the modified S-303 protocol are probably required and are under study at this time.

Chemicals That Require Photoactivation

Similar to the successful PI procedures applied to plasma and platelet products, treatment of red cells with a diverse group of photosensitizers has been extensively studied, although none have yet progressed to formal clinical assessment at any scale.

Dimethylmethylene blue (DMMB) is more hydrophobic and has a greater affinity for nucleic acids than methylene blue.[52-54] DMMB

(25 μmol/L) plus visible light has been shown to inactivate RNA and DNA viruses in aliquots of red cells and leukocytes. However, DMMB induced increased hemolysis (1%-40%).[53,54] As in other PI methods, the composition of the posttreatment storage solution seems to strongly affect the integrity of the red cells after photochemical treatment.[55] No clinical trials using DMMB have been reported to date.

Positively charged porphyrins have also been used. For instance, treatment with mono-phenyl-tri-(N-methyl-4-pyridyl)-porphyrin has been shown to exhibit activity against bacteria and vesicular stomatitis virus, and treated red cells have demonstrated acceptable biochemical parameters, storage stability, and in-vivo recovery and survival in rhesus monkeys.[56] Unfortunately, its efficiency against non-cell-associated human immunodeficiency virus (HIV) and nonenveloped viruses is poor, and it induces increased hemolysis in human red cells.[57]

Flexible photosensitizer dyes have also been used. These dyes contain aromatic rings separated by single bonds capable of rotating when the photosensitizer is not firmly bound to a substrate. The major advantage of these dyes is that they potentially differentiate between molecules bound to nucleic acid and those not bound or attached to other moieties. Only the nucleic-acid-bound dye becomes fixed and rigid, a change that alters its light-adsorption reaction, so that upon light activation, it will induce alkylation and the release of reactive oxygen species (ROS). When the unbound dye is illuminated, the dye absorbs the photon energy and dissipates it as heat energy without generating undesirable ROS. One such flexible, nucleic-acid-intercalating compound is thiopyrylium (TP) dye, with a strong affinity for nucleic acids but also for red cell membranes. It has been combined with dipyrimadole (DP), a competitive inhibitor of red cell membrane binding, to minimize the ability of TP to damage the red cell membrane through ROS production.[58] DP is an antioxidant that has been shown to reduce the photochemical damage of red cells and inhibit platelet aggregation. Structurally, DP resembles TP and seems to partially block the binding of TP to the red cell membrane. TP/DP has shown marked PI activity on bacteria (5 to 7 $\log_{10}$) and viruses, including HIV (>6 $\log_{10}$).[59] Like DMMB, the composition of the posttreatment storage solution seems to be crucial in the maintenance of the osmotic pressure between the extracellular and intracellular spaces after PI treatment.[60] As for other photoinactivation methods, rapid potassium leakage occurred in phototreated samples, a change that could result in increased ATP usage and increased hemolysis in some additive solutions, suggesting that DP is not sufficient to prevent TP binding to the red cell membrane.[59] No clinical trials have been reported to date.

Another flexible photosensitizer dye is thiazole orange (TO). TO is an asymmetrical intercalating cyanine dye that acts as a photosensitizer only when bound to nucleic acids.[61] Because only a minor fraction of TO is bound to red cells, a quencher is not required. TO has been shown to reduce viral loads from 5 to 7 $\log_{10}$ of tested viruses and 2 to 7 $\log_{10}$ of tested bacteria.[59,61] Forty-two-day stored red cells exhibited slightly increased hemolysis, increased potassium efflux, and similar levels of ATP when compared with control red cells.[61] No clinical trials using TO have been reported to date.

A riboflavin-based photoinactivation protocol for red cells shows promise. This is an approach that has already been successfully applied to PI in plasma and platelets.[62-65] This technology, Mirasol (CaridianBCT, Lakewood, CO), involves the addition of a final concentration of 50 mmol/L riboflavin (Fig 4-1) to washed red cell concentrates. Following association of riboflavin with the nucleic acid, and activation with blue light (447 to 470 nm light with a peak at 450 nm), a photochemical reaction modifies guanine residues and thus prevents nucleic acid replication.[62] More recently, the combination of 500 mmol/L riboflavin and ultraviolet (UV) light (280 to 350 nm with a peak at 313 nm) in PI of whole blood has resulted in effective PI in vitro and in vivo in animal models.[66] This approach yields acceptable levels of PI at maximum light intensities and maintains acceptable in-vitro levels of ATP concentration in red cells and platelets.[67] Notably, riboflavin and UV light treatment of whole blood has been shown to cause in-vitro leukocyte inactivation at doses as low as 33 and 44 J/mL, which prevents alloimmunization to platelet transfusion and cardiac transplants in rat models.[68] In-vivo results with components treated at 33 J/mL, using a xenogeneic model of GVHD, were compared with those for untreated components. Mice were injected with treated and untreated peripheral blood mononuclear cells (PBMCs). Those injected with untreated PBMCs exhibited decreased hematocrit, increased human $CD45^+$ cell engraftment, and increased levels of human IgG, IgM, and interferon when compared to those that received treated PBMCs.[67] Phase I trials of treated whole blood are under way to test the impact of Mirasol technology on leukocyte inactivation in red cells, platelets, and plasma proteins.

What Is the Future of Red Cell and Whole Blood Pathogen Inactivation?

In considering the potential use of PI for red cells and whole blood, it is worth highlighting that the currently used PI technologies have effectively eliminated the recognized infectious risks of commercial pooled plasma protein fractions for the established pathogens of concern. In addition, certain technologies (eg, pooled solvent/detergent-treated plasma and methylene-blue-treated fresh frozen plasma) are used for selected patients in some countries, despite some impact on hemostatic function. Reductions in the efficacy of red cell units might be accepted in exchange for the benefits of eliminating pathogens.

The risk of infectious transmission by red cell transfusion has dramatically decreased in the developed world as a result of the application of state-of-the-art technologies related to red cell collection, filtration, and storage. However, pathogen transmission remains a concern in red cell transfusion to chronically transfused patients, such as patients with thalassemia, where the prevalence of TT virus infection has been described as higher than in the nontransfused population,[69] and to patients in the developing world, as illustrated by the transmission risk of HHV-8.[70] Further, there will always be some risk of an emerging pathogen, or a pathogen whose incidence is underestimated and for which no test is yet available. Also, PI technologies have been shown to be capable of preventing TA-GVHD and possibly alloimmunization, replacing the need for irradiation (and potentially, leukocyte filtration) of blood components for susceptible patients. Hence, the application of PI technologies to red cells or whole blood has many attractions, particularly if these technologies can be applied to whole blood before component production.

Ideally, of course, PI technologies should inactivate pathogens (and leukocytes) in blood and its components without impairing the biologic functions for which they are being transfused. In the absence of this ideal, what loss of function is acceptable? To date, transfusion medicine has largely focused on poststorage red cell in-vivo recovery and survival as the primary measure of acceptability. Recent retrospective data have suggested that transfusion of red cells after prolonged storage may induce harm. While the possible deleterious effect of storage on red cells is currently undergoing analysis in at least two randomized trials, there has been a revitalization of interest in understanding red cell physiology, and, above all, in its interaction with the endothelium and in-vivo oxygen delivery.

Although considerable progress has been made in the development of S-303 and riboflavin for PI in red cells and whole blood, the development of these procedures is still in its infancy. The final question is this: Even after these newer DNA-targeted PI technologies pass the increasingly stringent regulatory requirements, will the health-care system pay the premium for safer blood? Certainly, health policy-makers will have to decide based on specific situations. The appearance of HIV in the 1980s completely changed the field of blood banking; the threat of another emergent pathogen of similar virulence may change it again.

Acknowledgments

The author wishes to thank Margaret O'Leary for her helpful comments and edits on the text as well as Larry Corash from Cerus Corporation and Ray Goodrich from CaridianBCT Biotechnologies for providing publication updates.

References

1. Ruhl H, Bein G, Sachs UJ. Transfusion-associated graft-versus-host disease. Transfus Med Rev 2009;23:62-71.
2. Hirayama J, Abe H, Azuma H, Ikeda H. Leakage of potassium from red blood cells following gamma ray irradiation in the presence of dipyridamole, trolox, human plasma or mannitol. Biol Pharm Bull 2005;28:1318-20.
3. Mintz PD, Wehrli G. Irradiation eradication and pathogen reduction. Ceasing cesium irradiation of blood products. Bone Marrow Transplant 2009;44:205-11.
4. Fergusson D, Khanna MP, Tinmouth A, Hebert PC. Transfusion of leukoreduced red blood cells may decrease postoperative infections: Two meta-analyses of randomized controlled trials. Can J Anaesth 2004;51:417-24.
5. Zhang X, Araki N, Ito K. Post-transfusion alloimmunization to granulocytes and platelets in Japanese patients as determined by the MPHA method. Transfus Apher Sci 2001;25:163-72.
6. Frietsch T, Karger R, Scholer M, et al. Leukodepletion of autologous whole blood has no impact on perioperative infection rate and length of hospital stay. Transfusion 2008;48:2133-42.

7. Hendrickson JE, Hillyer CD. Noninfectious serious hazards of transfusion. Anesth Analg 2009;108:759-69.
8. Marik PE. The hazards of blood transfusion. Br J Hosp Med (Lond) 2009; 70:12-15.
9. Goodnough LT. Risks of blood transfusion. Anesthesiol Clin North America 2005;23:241-52.
10. McClaskey J, Xu M, Snyder EL, Tormey CA. Clinical trials for pathogen reduction in transfusion medicine: A review. Transfus Apher Sci 2009;41:217-25.
11. Wu YY, Snyder EL. Safety of the blood supply: Role of pathogen reduction. Blood Rev 2003;17:111-22.
12. Centers for Disease Control and Prevention. Red blood cell transfusions contaminated with *Yersinia enterocolitica*—United States, 1991-1996, and initiation of a national study to detect bacteria-associated transfusion reactions. MMWR Morb Mortal Wkly Rep 1997;46:553-5.
13. Leclercq A, Martin L, Vergnes ML, et al. Fatal *Yersinia enterocolitica* biotype 4 serovar O:3 sepsis after red blood cell transfusion. Transfusion 2005;45: 814-18.
14. Polizzotto MN, Neo H, Spelman D, et al. *Streptococcus pneumoniae* septicemia associated with red blood cell transfusion. Transfusion 2008;48:1520-1.
15. AuBuchon JP, Dzik WH. Survival of *Loa loa* in banked blood. Lancet 1983; 1:647-8.
16. Bowden RA, Slichter SJ, Sayers M, et al. A comparison of filtered leukocyte-reduced and cytomegalovirus (CMV) seronegative blood products for the prevention of transfusion-associated CMV infection after marrow transplant. Blood 1995;86:3598-603.
17. Narvios AB, de Lima M, Shah H, Lichtiger B. Transfusion of leukoreduced cellular blood components from cytomegalovirus-unscreened donors in allogeneic hematopoietic transplant recipients: Analysis of 72 recipients. Bone Marrow Transplant 2005;36:499-501.
18. Nichols WG, Price TH, Gooley T, et al. Transfusion-transmitted cytomegalovirus infection after receipt of leukoreduced blood products. Blood 2003; 101:4195-200.
19. Cesaire R, Kerob-Bauchet B, Bourdonne O, et al. Evaluation of HTLV-I removal by filtration of blood cell components in a routine setting. Transfusion 2004;44:42-8.
20. Laperche S, Worms B, Pillonel J. Blood safety strategies for human T-cell lymphotropic virus in Europe. Vox Sang 2009;96:104-10.
21. Pennington J, Taylor GP, Sutherland J, et al. Persistence of HTLV-I in blood components after leukocyte depletion. Blood 2002;100:677-81.
22. Seghatchian J. Universal leucodepletion: An overview of some unresolved issues and the highlights of lessons learned. Transfus Apher Sci 2003;29:105-17.
23. Rebulla P, Porretti L, Bertolini F, et al. White cell-reduced red cells prepared by filtration: A critical evaluation of current filters and methods for counting residual white cells. Transfusion 1993;33:128-33.
24. AuBuchon JP, Cancelas JA, Herschel L, et al. In vitro and in vivo evaluation of LEUKOSEP HRC-600-C leukoreduction filtration system for red cells. Transfusion 2006;46:1311-15.

25. Gregori L, Gurgel PV, Lathrop JT, et al. Reduction in infectivity of endogenous transmissible spongiform encephalopathies present in blood by adsorption to selective affinity resins. Lancet 2006;368:2226-30.
26. Gregori L, Lambert BC, Gurgel PV, et al. Reduction of transmissible spongiform encephalopathy infectivity from human red blood cells with prion protein affinity ligands. Transfusion 2006;46:1152-61.
27. Bégué SS, Sumian C, Walicka I. Storage study of red blood cells treated with the Macopharma P-CAPT prion removal filter (abstract). Transfus Med 2006; 16(Suppl 1):36.
28. Cancelas J, Rugg N, Pratt PG, Worsham DN, et al. P-Capt filtered RBC maintain adequate hematological, biochemical and in vivo recovery levels after storage (abstract). Transfusion 2009;49(Suppl):37A-38A.
29. Davenport RD, Judd W, Downs T, Pehta JC, et al. The P-Capt prion filter does not alter red cell antigens (abstract). Transfusion 2009;49(Suppl):104A-105A.
30. Sowemino-Coker SO, Demczyk CA, Andrade F, Baker CA. Evaluation of removal of prion infectivity from red blood cells with prion reduction filters using a new rapid and highly sensitive cell culture-based infectivity assay. Transfusion 2010;50:980-8.
31. Purmal A, Valeri CR, Dzik W, et al. Process for the preparation of pathogen-inactivated RBC concentrates by using PEN110 chemistry: Preclinical studies. Transfusion 2002;42:139-45.
32. Lazo A, Tassello J, Jayarama V, et al. Broad-spectrum virus reduction in red cell concentrates using INACTINE PEN110 chemistry. Vox Sang 2002;83: 313-23.
33. AuBuchon JP, Pickard CA, Herschel LH, et al. Production of pathogen-inactivated RBC concentrates using PEN110 chemistry: A Phase I clinical study. Transfusion 2002;42:146-52.
34. Zavizion B, Serebryanik D, Chapman J, et al. Inactivation of Gram-negative and Gram-positive bacteria in red cell concentrates using INACTINE PEN110 chemistry. Vox Sang 2004;87:143-9.
35. Ohagen A, Gibaja V, Horrigan J, et al. Induction of latent human cytomegalovirus by conventional gamma irradiation and prevention by treatment with INACTINE PEN110. Vox Sang 2004;87:1-9.
36. Zavizion B, Pereira M, de Melo Jorge M, et al. Inactivation of protozoan parasites in red blood cells using INACTINE PEN110 chemistry. Transfusion 2004;44:731-8.
37. Aytay S, Ohagen A, Busch MR, et al. Development of a sensitive PCR inhibition method to demonstrate HBV nucleic acid inactivation. Transfusion 2004;44:476-84.
38. Zavizion B, Purmal A, Chapman J, Alford B. Inactivation of mycoplasma species in blood by INACTINE PEN110 process. Transfusion 2004;44:286-93.
39. Fast LD, Semple JW, DiLeone G, et al. Inhibition of xenogeneic GVHD by PEN110 treatment of donor human PBMNCs. Transfusion 2004;44:282-5.
40. Mather T, Takeda T, Tassello J, et al. West Nile virus in blood: Stability, distribution, and susceptibility to PEN110 inactivation. Transfusion 2003;43: 1029-37.

41. Jayarama V, Marcello J, Ohagen A, et al. Development of models and detection methods for different forms of cytomegalovirus for the evaluation of viral inactivation agents. Transfusion 2006;46:1580-8.
42. Chapman JR, Moore K, Butterworth BE. Pathogen inactivation of RBCs: PEN110 reproductive toxicology studies. Transfusion 2003;43:1386-93.
43. Zavizion B, Serebryanik D, Serebryanik I, et al. Prevention of *Yersinia enterocolitica, Pseudomonas fluorescens,* and *Pseudomonas putida* outgrowth in deliberately inoculated blood by a novel pathogen-reduction process. Transfusion 2003;43:135-42.
44. Chapman J. Pathogen inactivation of red cell concentrates using Inactine chemistry. Transfus Apher Sci 2001;25:191-2.
45. Rios JA, Hambleton J, Viele M, et al. Viability of red cells prepared with S-303 pathogen inactivation treatment. Transfusion 2006;46:1778-86.
46. Mufti NA, Erickson AC, North AK, et al. Treatment of whole blood (WB) and red blood cells (RBC) with S-303 inactivates pathogens and retains in vitro quality of stored RBC. Biologicals 2010;38:14-19.
47. Benjamin RJ, McCullough J, Mintz PD, et al. Therapeutic efficacy and safety of red blood cells treated with a chemical process (S-303) for pathogen inactivation: A Phase III clinical trial in cardiac surgery patients. Transfusion 2005;45:1739-49.
48. Corash L. Inactivation of infectious pathogens in labile blood components: Meeting the challenge. Transfus Clin Biol 2001;8:138-45.
49. Conlan MGG, Garraty G, Castro G, et al. Antibodies to S-303 treated red blood cells prepared with the original treatment process for pathogen inactivation do not react with red blood cells prepared with a modified S-303 treatment process (abstract). Blood 2005;106:430.
50. Cancelas JA, Dumont L, Herschel L, et al. A randomized, controlled, 2-period crossover study of recovery and lifespan of radiolabeled autologous 35-day old red blood cells prepared with a modified S-303 treatment for pathogen inactivation (abstract). Presented at the International Society of Blood Transfusion International Congress, Macao, June 7-12, 2008.
51. Skripchenko AA, Wagner SJ. Inactivation of WBCs in RBC suspensions by photoactive phenothiazine dyes: Comparison of dimethylmethylene blue and MB. Transfusion 2000;40:968-75.
52. Wagner SJ. Virus inactivation in blood components by photoactive phenothiazine dyes. Transfus Med Rev 2002;16:61-6.
53. Wagner SJ, Skripchenko A, Robinette D, et al. The use of dimethylmethylene blue for virus photoinactivation of red cell suspensions. Dev Biol (Basel) 2000;102:125-9.
54. Wagner SJ, Skripchenko A. Investigation of photosensitizing dyes for pathogen reduction in red cell suspensions. Biotech Histochem 2003;78:171-7.
55. Trannoy LL, Lagerberg JW, Dubbelman TM, et al. Positively charged porphyrins: A new series of photosensitizers for sterilization of RBCs. Transfusion 2004;44:1186-96.
56. Trannoy LL, Terpstra FG, de Korte D, et al. Differential sensitivities of pathogens in red cell concentrates to Tri-P(4)-photoinactivation. Vox Sang 2006; 91:111-18.

57. Besselink GA, van Engelenburg FA, Ebbing IG, et al. Additive effects of dipyridamole and Trolox in protecting human red cells during photodynamic treatment. Vox Sang 2003;85:25-30.
58. Wagner SJ, Skripchenko A, Cincotta L, et al. Use of a flexible thiopyrylium photosensitizer and competitive inhibitor for pathogen reduction of viruses and bacteria with retention of red cell storage properties. Transfusion 2005; 45:752-60.
59. Besselink GA, Ebbing IG, Hilarius PM, et al. Composition of the additive solution affects red blood cell integrity after photodynamic treatment. Vox Sang 2003;85:183-9.
60. Skripchenko A, Wagner SJ, Thompson-Montgomery D, Awatefe H. Thiazole orange, a DNA-binding photosensitizer with flexible structure, can inactivate pathogens in red blood cell suspensions while maintaining red cell storage properties. Transfusion 2006;46:213-19.
61. Goodrich RP. The use of riboflavin for the inactivation of pathogens in blood products. Vox Sang 2000;78(Suppl 2):211-15.
62. Cardo LJ, Rentas FJ, Ketchum L, et al. Pathogen inactivation of *Leishmania donovani infantum* in plasma and platelet concentrates using riboflavin and ultraviolet light. Vox Sang 2006;90:85-91.
63. Cardo LJ, Salata J, Mendez J, et al. Pathogen inactivation of *Trypanosoma cruzi* in plasma and platelet concentrates using riboflavin and ultraviolet light. Transfus Apher Sci 2007;37:131-7.
64. Ruane PH, Edrich R, Gampp D, et al. Photochemical inactivation of selected viruses and bacteria in platelet concentrates using riboflavin and light. Transfusion 2004;44:877-85.
65. Goodrich RP, Murthy KK, Doane SK, et al. Evaluation of potential immune response and in vivo survival of riboflavin-ultraviolet light-treated red blood cells in baboons. Transfusion 2009;49:64-74.
66. Goodrich RP, Doane S, Reddy HL. Design and development of a method for the reduction of infectious pathogen load and inactivation of white blood cells in whole blood products. Biologicals 2010;38:20-30.
67. Asano H, Lee CY, Fox-Talbot K, et al. Treatment with riboflavin and ultraviolet light prevents alloimmunization to platelet transfusions and cardiac transplants. Transplantation 2007;84:1174-82.
68. Ozyurek E, Ergunay K, Kuskonmaz B, et al. Transfusion-transmitted virus prevalence in Turkish patients with thalassemia. Pediatr Hematol Oncol 2006;23:347-53.
69. Hladik W, Dollard SC, Mermin J, et al. Transmission of human herpesvirus 8 by blood transfusion. N Engl J Med 2006;355:1331-8.
70. Cerus Corporation reports positive outcome of phase 1 clinical trial of intercept red blood cells (press release, February 8, 2010). Concord, CA: Cerus Corp, 2010.

In: AuBuchon JP, Prowse CV, eds.
Pathogen Inactivation: The Penultimate Paradigm Shift
Bethesda, MD: AABB Press, 2010

5

Pathogen Inactivation of Plasma and Cryoprecipitate

BJARTE G. SOLHEIM, MD, PHD, MHA,
AND PETER HELLSTERN, MD

PATHOGEN INACTIVATION (PI) OF PLASMA CAN BE performed on either single plasma units or pooled plasma units. Three technologies have been granted the Conformité Européenne (CE) mark and are currently used for PI of single plasma units in blood banks. Thus far, the US Food and Drug Administration (FDA) has approved these technologies in the United States only for use in clinical trials. In other geographic regions, some are approved for use,

---

Bjarte G. Solheim, MD, PhD, MHA, Professor Emeritus, Institute of Immunology, Oslo University Hospital—Rikshospitalet and University of Oslo, Oslo, Norway, and Peter Hellstern, MD, Director and Professor, Institute of Hemostaseology and Transfusion Medicine, Academic City Hospital Ludwigshafen, Ludwigshafen, Germany

The authors have disclosed no conflicts of interest.

others not. Pooled biopharmaceutical PI plasma (60-360 L) is licensed as medicine in many countries. PI technology for small plasma pools (5-10 L) has been developed for use in blood banks in resource-limited countries.

Pathogen-Inactivation Technologies for Plasma

Currently, only two fundamentally different approaches to PI of plasma are in use: solvent/detergent (SD) treatment to disrupt lipid-enveloped pathogens, or the addition of nucleic-acid-binding heterocyclic sensitizers that inactivate DNA/RNA upon light exposure (photosensitizers). Two other methods that have been described but not further developed are pasteurization (1992) and nanofiltration (2003).[1,2]

Solvent/Detergent Treatment

SD treatment was introduced in 1986.[3] This method is very robust[4] and removes infectivity by effectively disrupting the membranes of lipid-enveloped viruses, cells, and most protozoa, although its efficacy with respect to bacteria is variable, and it is ineffective against non-lipid-enveloped viruses. It is the most widely used and best validated PI technology; more than 60 million doses of SD-treated, pooled, fractionated plasma proteins have been transfused without any report of transmission of enveloped viruses. The method was adapted for PI of plasma in 1991 by Horowitz et al in the United States and Hellstern et al in Germany.[5,6] For plasma and most plasma proteins, a combination of 1% tri-(N-butyl)-phosphate (TNBP) and 1% polyoxyethylene-p-t-octylphenol (Triton X-100) for 4 hours at 30 to 31 C is applied to ensure PI.[7] TNBP is used alone in some protocols for PI and acts as an organic solvent to remove lipids from the pathogen membranes. Triton X-100 is a nonionic detergent that stabilizes TNBP and disrupts lipid bilayers, easing the extraction of lipids.[7] SD treatment was first licensed for clotting factors in the second half of the 1980s and has been in use for the treatment of plasma since 1991.[5,6] SD treatment is preceded by filtration with a 1-μm filter to remove cells and followed by a final sterile filtration step involving filtration with a 0.2-µm filter and aseptic filling into bags/vials.

The inactivation rate of enveloped viruses in plasma is extremely high, and virus is below detection levels (>6 log) within 2 minutes,[4] except for vaccinia virus, which shows a relative resistance[8] but which nevertheless can be inactivated according to the protocol mentioned above with TNBP and Triton X-100 within 10 minutes (T.-E. Svae, Octapharma, personal communication). To date, all tested enveloped viruses, including recently emerging viruses such as West Nile virus, chikungunya virus, new influenza strains, and severe acute respiratory syndrome coronavirus, can be inactivated. No second PI step is available for pooled plasma, but immune antibodies that are usually naturally present in a plasma pool can protect against infection with the most commonly encountered nonenveloped viruses such as hepatitis A virus and parvovirus B19.[9,10] Safety regulations therefore involve the setting of upper limits for hepatitis A and parvovirus B19 virus particle content in a pool and minimum titers for the corresponding antibodies.

SD-treated, pooled fresh frozen plasma (FFP; 100-1520 donations) was introduced in Europe in 1991, with Octaplas (Octapharma AG, Lachen, Switzerland) as the leading product. Octaplas is a licensed biopharmaceutical product in 29 countries worldwide (including Canada and Mexico in North America). With licensure from Octapharma AG, SD plasma is produced in Italy and France. In France the batch size is limited to 60 L (100 plasmapheresis units). A total of over 6.5 million units of SD-treated plasma have been transfused to date. Bioplasma FDP (fresh human plasma: lyophilized powder for intravenous infusion; manufactured by National Bioproducts Institute, Pinetown, South Africa) is an ABO-independent, universal SD plasma that has been in production for more than 12 years under license from Octapharma AG, with more than 400,000 units transfused in South Africa.[11] In the United States, pooled SD plasma (PLAS+SD, from 500-2500 donations) was produced by Vitex (Watertown, MA) and licensed in the second half of the 1990s but later withdrawn from the market.[11] (This withdrawal was primarily for commercial reasons, but concerns had also arisen about thrombogenicity of the product because of significant reduction in antithrombogenic proteins.) After SD treatment of FFP, products are normally frozen in 200-mL plastic bags; Bioplasma FDP, however, is lyophilized.

OctaplasLG is an SD plasma in which a chromatographic step with a specific prion-binding ligand gel is combined with reduced SD treatment time of 1 to 1.5 hours.[12] The combination of prion ligand gel and the prion reduction already obtained through the SD treatment process[13] results in >5 log reduction of abnormal prion protein (PrP^{Sc}). OctaplasLG, expected to replace the original Octaplas, is so far licensed in Germany and Australia, but the regulatory procedure is ongoing in other countries in Europe. In some of these countries there has been a request for confirmatory studies on the claimed prion removal capacity. These studies are about to be completed (T-E. Svae, Octapharma, personal communication). The ABO-independent, universal SD plasma Uniplas (working title) was developed by Octapharma using proportional pooling of A, B, and AB plasma. Uniplas has been used successfully in clinical trials in Europe in cardiac surgery and liver resection[14-16] and is now in the final stages of licensing.

Burnouf and collaborators introduced "minipool" (5-10 L) SD treatment suitable for resource-limited countries in 2006.[17,18] They substituted Triton X-100 with Triton X-45, which seems as effective as Triton X-100 but causes less inactivation of plasmin inhibitor (synonym: α_2-antiplasmin). Triton X-45 and X- 100 differ in molecular mass, the former having only five ethylene oxide groups, and the latter, nine to ten groups. This difference in molecular mass suggests that these two nonionic detergents may differently affect the conformation (and activity) of plasmin inhibitor.[19] The application of a closed multibag system, different filters, and oil extraction procedures can, in addition to the small volume, be of importance for reduced inactivation of plasmin inhibitor.

Photosensitizers

Heterocyclic sensitizers with affinity for nucleic acids inactivate pathogens upon exposure to light [visible or ultraviolet (UV)]. Once bound to the nucleic acids of viruses, bacteria, parasites, or cells, exposure to light will either cause direct damage to the nucleic acids or induce cross-links between nucleic acids, blocking DNA and RNA dependent function.

Methylene Blue/Light Treatment

The virus inactivating activity of illuminated phenothiazines had already been recognized by the early 1930s.[20] Methylene blue (MB) is a positively charged phenothiazine dye that has a high affinity for the negatively charged nucleic acid guanine, and some binding also occurs in proteins and lipids. MB most likely interacts with guanine through intercalative binding and produces singlet oxygen-mediated damage when irradiated with visible light for about 30 minutes.[21] MB light treatment is effective against enveloped and some nonenveloped viruses, but MB may be unable to inactivate intracellular pathogens or leukocytes fully, because it cannot permeate plasma membranes effectively.[7,11]

MB/light-treated plasma (MB plasma) is the second most commonly used PI plasma, and more than 4 million units have been used clinically in Germany, Belgium, France, Greece, Italy, Spain, Switzerland, and the United Kingdom. The original Springe protocol (DRK-Blutspendedienst Niedersachsen, Institut Springe, Germany) involved industrial PI of single plasma units. This process was in use for more than a decade in Germany and Switzerland.[22,23] A similar factory-based method was introduced by Grifols (Barcelona, Spain), involving in this case filtration instead of the freeze-thaw step used in the Springe protocol for leukocyte removal. This method is still in use in Spain. Baxter and Macopharma (Tourcoing, France) modified the MB/light treatment of plasma for use in blood centers, improving the method by introducing a 0.65-µm plasma filter and a device to remove more than 90% of MB and its photoproducts without significant additional loss of coagulation factors. Only the Macopharma system (Theraflex MB-Plasma system) is currently available for use in blood banks.[11] The system has been granted the CE mark and is used to prepare single-donor PI plasma in house at a number of blood banks in Europe. In Germany, the Paul Ehrlich Institute (Frankfurt, Germany) has granted authorization to manufacture and sell plasma inactivated using the Theraflex MB-Plasma system.

Psoralen/Ultraviolet Light Treatment

Psoralens are active furocouramine compounds isolated from plants and have been known as photosensitizers since ancient times.[7]

Cerus (Concord, CA) selected a synthetic psoralen, amotosalen hydrochloric acid (S-59), for commercial development for PI because it crosses plasma membranes efficiently and demonstrates excellent protection against pathogens.[7] It is activated by ultraviolet A (UVA) light.

After addition to plasma, S-59 intercalates almost instantly with the helical region of single or double-stranded DNA and RNA. UVA light induces a covalent bond between S-59 and pyrimidine; after continued UVA light exposure, a second bond is generated that cross-links double-stranded structures, while single-stranded structures are cross-linked in loops. S-59/UVA-light treatment efficiently inactivates a broad spectrum of enveloped viruses, bacteria, protozoa, and residual leukocytes, but its effect on nonenveloped viruses is more variable.[7,24]

For PI of plasma with S-59 and UVA illumination (315-400 nm for about 4 minutes), Cerus has developed the Intercept Blood System, which uses a compound adsorption device (CAD) filter to remove residual S-59 and metabolites. The system can also be used for platelets. In Europe it was granted the CE mark for PI of plasma in 2006. It has an input volume of 385-650 mL of plasma and has been implemented under good manufacturing practice conditions in blood banks. About 10,000 plasma portions have been pathogen inactivated to date (mostly apheresis plasma, but also some representing a pool of three single plasma units from recovered blood).

Riboflavin/Light Treatment

Vitamin B2, riboflavin (RF), is classified "generally recognized as safe" by the FDA in the United States despite its phototoxic targeting of nucleic acids. RF and its photoproducts are present in a wide range of common foods and natural products. Along with its photoproducts and catabolites, RF is also detectable in normal blood, which suggests it may be ubiquitous.[25]

The phototoxic PI effect of RF involves both oxygen-dependent processes (formation of free radicals) and oxygen-independent processes (electron transfer). These processes damage guanine and may form adducts of thymine and adenine.[26,27] RF/light treatment has proven effective against a range of pathogens, including bacteria, enveloped viruses, protozoa, leukocytes, and some nonenveloped viruses.[25]

The Mirasol system for the RF/light treatment of blood components was developed by Navigant Biotechnologies (now Caridian-BCT Biotechnologies, Lakewood, CO). For PI of plasma the system applies UV light (285-365 nm, a spectrum that includes UVA and UVB) with an illumination time of 6 to 7 minutes.[27] The system is similar to Intercept except that it does not use a CAD, because RF, its photoproducts, and catabolites are naturally present in blood. After successful clinical trials, the Mirasol system was CE marked for PI of plasma in 2008, and it is currently being introduced to blood banks in Europe.

Toxicity

Solvent/Detergent

Oil extraction and chromatographic steps are applied to remove SD reagents from plasma subsequent to PI. The European Pharmacopoeia (6.2, July 2008:1646) requires residual amounts in SD plasma to be <2 µg/mL TNBP and <5 µg/mL Triton X-100 (in most batches of Octaplas, SD reagents are below the detectable level which is 0.5 and 1 µg/mL respectively). In the minipool procedure, TNBP is reduced to <10 parts per million for Triton X-100 and <50 parts per million for Triton X-45.[18] These values are far below both toxicity levels and ambient environmental exposures in industrialized societies.[7] The safety of the SD treatment has further been demonstrated by the more than 6.5 million units of SD plasma and >60 million units of SD-treated plasma proteins that have been transfused without report of toxicity or neoantigenicity.

Methylene Blue

MB is low in toxicity. Intravenous doses of 1 to 5 mgMB/kg have been administered in clinical situations without report of serious adverse events. A unit of MB plasma represents 0.0012 mgMB/kg for an adult and is reduced further to 0.00012 mg MB/kg by the filtration step.[11] In addition, Macopharma has performed a formal toxicology study as part of the German licensure. After transfusion of >4 million units MB PI plasma, no toxicity or neoantigenicity from various residual intercalated proteins after MB light treatment has been reported. On a theoretical level, however, long-term side effects cannot be ruled out completely.[28,29]

Psoralen (S-59 or Amotosalen)

Extensive studies from the start of the planned introduction of Intercept-treated plasma for clinical use did not demonstrate any neoantigenicity or toxicologically relevant effects for S-59.[24] Additional reduction of the S-59 dose and its degradation products can be obtained through the introduction of the CAD.[30] Clinical experience with the transfusion of >400,000 units of platelets and >10,000 units of plasma treated with the Intercept system have not revealed any toxicity or neoantigenicity. Some reaction of S-59 with proteins and lipids does occur, however, so long-term side effects cannot be ruled out completely.[28,29]

Riboflavin

Riboflavin is a naturally occurring vitamin with a high safety profile. Its photoproducts and catabolites are naturally present and detectable in normal blood. No device has therefore been introduced to remove RF and its photoproducts after Mirasol treatment of plasma. The need for additional research nevertheless remains, because the level of RF photoproducts is considerably higher in Mirasol-treated blood components than in natural blood. Introduction of Mirasol-treated plasma in clinics should therefore be closely monitored by hemovigilance systems.

Impact of PI on Plasma Protein Concentrations and Functions

PI invariably affects relevant proteins in transfusion plasma. A compromise must therefore be found between the extent of microbial kill and the effect on labile plasma proteins such as coagulation factors. The activity of Factor VIII, the most labile of coagulation factors, is frequently used to assess the quality of PI processes. The four established PI procedures entail the loss of 20% to 30% of Factor VIII activity, and less than 20% for most other coagulation factors or inhibitors except as noted below[29] and in Table 5-1. Considering the wide normal range (50%-200%) for coagulation factors, reductions on this scale are not regarded as clinically significant. Moreover, the quality of the FFP used for PI may vary widely depending on a number of factors. For example, optimal freezing and storage at temperatures <–20 C is important. Other quality-related factors include the source of the plasma or the way in which the recovered plasma was handled. Apheresis plasma frozen promptly after donation is superior, followed by recovered plasma frozen within 4 hours and plasma frozen within 15 hours. Delayed or slow freezing of plasma reduces both coagulation factor and protease inhibitor activities; repeated thawing/freezing particularly affects coagulation Factors V, VIII, and XI.[41,42] Finally, the ABO blood group of the plasma donor influences the concentration of Factor VIII and von Willebrand factor (VWF) significantly.

Solvent/Detergent

SD treatment is the only current technology suitable for PI of pooled plasma. Pooling in batches of 60 to 380 L allows for the production of standardized biopharmaceutical products with extensive in-process control and uniform concentrations of plasma proteins, unlike the wide variations naturally found in single-donor plasma. Pooling also dilutes and in some instances neutralizes antibodies and allergens and allows the production of ABO-independent universal plasma (Bioplasma FDP and Uniplas). To reduce the risk of emerging transfusion-transmitted infections, a pool size of 60 to 380 L is now used for SD plasma, which is much smaller than the 4000 to 30,000 L used for PI fractionated plasma proteins.

SD treatment targets lipids and so has little direct effect on transfusion-relevant proteins in plasma. Differences between in-production processes demonstrated strikingly lower protein S, plasmin inhibitor, plasminogen activator inhibitor, and antitrypsin activities in PLAS+SD than in Octaplas, where only plasmin inhibitor activity is reduced, in this case to ~27% of normal levels.[43-45] In the new Octa-

Table 5-1. Impact of Pathogen Inactivation and Inevitable Dilution, Freezing, and Thawing on Hemostasis in Therapeutic Plasma*

	Treatment			
Effects	**SD (Octaplas)**	**MB Light**	**Psoralen UV Light (Intercept)**	**Riboflavin UV Light (Mirasol)**
General effects from dilution, freezing, and thawing (decrease)	10%-25%†	10%-25%†	10%-25%†	10%-25%†
Method-specific effects	Plasmin inhibitor: 76% decrease[31] (OctaplasLG: 37% decrease[32]) Protein S: 35% decrease[31]	Fibrinogen: 20%-39% decrease[33,34] Impaired fibrin thrombin generation and fibrin polymerization[35,36,37]	Fibrinogen: 11%-28% decrease[34,38,39]	Fibrinogen and Factors V, VII, IX, X: 30% decrease[40] Factors VIII, XI: 40% decrease[40]

*Absolute potencies are not shown because these depend strongly on the plasma submitted for pathogen inactivation.
†Factor VIII is the most labile coagulation factor, with a general in-process loss of up to 25%.
Manufacturers: Octaplas = Octapharma AG, Lachen, Switzerland; Intercept = Cerus Corp, Concord, CA; Mirasol = CaridianBCT, Lakewood, CO.
SD = solvent/detergent; MB = methylene blue; UV = ultraviolet.

plasLG, where incubation with SD reagents is reduced to 1 to 1.5 hours, the activity of plasmin inhibitors is increased to ~63%, and protein S activity is ~66%, despite introduction of the additional processing step with the prion-binding ligand.[32] Thus, in OctaplasLG all coagulation factors and inhibitors are above the accepted lower normal level of 50%. In minipool plasma, where Triton X-100 is substituted with Triton X-45, plasmin inhibitors and protein S are even less affected.[19]

Methylene Blue

MB/light treatment of plasma particularly affects clottable fibrinogen, of which about 20% to 39% is lost.[11,33,34] This results in significantly prolonged fibrin polymerization time, which can be normalized, however, by admixture of 60% Octaplas.[35] Thrombin generation capacity is also impaired in MB plasma, but this had relatively little effect on the strength of clot as assessed by thromboelastography.[35-37]

Psoralen (S-59 or Amotosalen) and Riboflavin

For Intercept-treated plasma, a reduction has been reported in fibrinogen content from 11% to 28%.[34,38,39,46] In Mirasol-treated plasma fibrinogen, Factors V, VII, IX, and X are reduced by 30%, while VIII and XI are decreased by 32%.[40,47]

Clinical Studies and Experience with PI Plasma

Solvent/Detergent-Treated Plasma

At least 18 studies and retrospective analyses to examine the efficacy and tolerance of SD plasma, including two studies on universal SD plasma (Uniplas),[15,16] have been conducted, covering all indications for plasma (Table 5-2).[48-64] Four of these trials were designed as prospective randomized studies to compare SD plasma with standard FFP or MB plasma.[53-56] Although all of these studies involved

Table 5-2. Clinical Trials of Solvent/Detergent-Treated Plasma

Study Group	Design	Clinical Setting	Main Results
Hellstern et al (1993)[48]	Observational (n = 30)	Complex coagulopathy, massive transfusion	PT correction and increase in fibrinogen and AT
Inbal et al (1993)[49]	Observational (n = 8)	Hereditary deficiencies of Factors VII, X, and XI	Prevention or arrest of bleeding Normal half-life times of clotting factors
Solheim et al (1993)[50]	Observational: SD plasma (n = 43) vs FFP (n = 20)	Open-heart surgery	No clinical difference
Badoux et al (1998)[51]	Retrospective analysis: 894 recipients of 5064 SD plasma units	All indications for plasma	No severe adverse events
Horowitz, Pehta (1998)[52]	Observational: 396 treatment episodes, 164 patients	Severe coagulopathy (n = 85) Hereditary deficiencies of fibrinogen and Factors II, V, VII, X, XI, and XIII (n = 47) TTP (n = 32)	Prevention or arrest of bleeding in 87% TTP: no difference between SD plasma and FFP
Wieding et al (1999)[53]	Prospective, randomized (n = 71): SD plasma vs MB plasma	Cardiopulmonary bypass surgery	No clinical difference No increase in protein S and plasmin inhibitor levels after SD plasma

Williamson et al (1999)[54]	Prospective, randomized (n = 49): SD plasma vs FFP	Complex coagulopathy in liver disease or liver transplantation	Equal clinical efficacy and correction of coagulation parameters
Beck et al (2000)[55]	Prospective, randomized (n = 40): SD plasma vs FFP	Severe coagulopathy	Equal clinical efficacy and correction of coagulation parameters
Lerner et al (2000)[56]	Prospective, randomized (n = 45): SD plasma vs FFP	Prolonged PT from severe coagulopathy	No clinical difference No differences in correction of PT
Haubelt et al (2002)[57]	Prospective: SD plasma (n = 36) vs FFP (n = 31)	Severe coagulopathy after open-heart surgery	No clinical difference Pretreatment/posttreatment differences in protein S and plasmin inhibitor were lower after SD plasma
de Jonge et al (2002/2003)[58.59]	Retrospective analysis: SD plasma (n = 20) vs FFP (n = 21)	Coagulopathy in liver transplantation	No significant difference in total blood loss
Solheim et al (2003)[60]	Retrospective analysis (n = 208)	Liver transplantation	No particular problems with hyperfibrinolysis
Tollofsrud et al (2003)[15]	Observational: universal SD plasma (n = 36) vs SD plasma (n =19)	Open-heart surgery	No clinical difference; both plasma types hemostatic No adverse events
Solheim et al (2005)[16]	Prospective: universal SD plasma (n = 81)	Liver resection	Clinically efficient No adverse events, including hemolysis

(Continued)

Table 5-2. Clinical Trials of Solvent/Detergent-Treated Plasma (Continued)

Study Group	Design	Clinical Setting	Main Results
Chekrizova, Murphy (2006)[61]	Observational: 41 neonates, 15 children, 55 adults	Severe coagulopathy, liver disease, obstetric and gynecologic emergencies	Significant decreases in aPTT and PT No adverse reactions
McCarthy (2006)[62]	Retrospective analysis: SD plasma (n = 35) vs FFP (n = 62) vs cryo-poor plasma (n = 48)	TTP, plasma exchange	Significantly higher response rate with SD plasma compared with cryo-poor plasma (91% vs 70%; p = 0.02) No allergic reactions under SD plasma
Santagostino et al (2006)[63]	Observational (n = 17)	Hereditary deficiencies of fibrinogen and Factors V, VIII, X, XI 16 elective procedures, 1 surgical emergency	100% clinical efficacy after prolonged treatment with higher doses necessary in 3 cases Normal half-life times of Factors V, VIII, X
Scully et al (2007)[64]	Observational: 50 plasma exchange episodes in 32 patients; SD plasma vs cryosupernatant vs cryosupernatant followed by SD plasma	TTP, plasma exchange	Equal clinical efficacy Allergic and citrate reactions reduced by 50% in the SD-plasma-only group

PT = prothrombin time; AT = antithrombin; SD = solvent/detergent; FFP = fresh frozen plasma; TTP = thrombotic thrombocytopenic purpura; MB = methylene blue; aPTT = activated partial thromboplastin time.

relatively small numbers of cases and so lack the statistical power to detect small differences, they clearly show that reduced coagulation factor and inhibitor levels caused by SD treatment did not result in any significant impairment of clinical efficacy and tolerance. Concerns about the low levels of plasmin inhibitor, protein S, or antitrypsin activity in SD plasma[65-68] have not been confirmed in clinical studies, and observations in support of thrombosis or hyperfibrinolytic bleeding triggered by low protein S or plasmin inhibitor potencies in Octaplas have not withstood critical revision (see Chapter 7).[42,59,60,64,69] The fact that SD plasma is a clear, standardized solution with a defined constant volume has made it particularly popular among anesthesiologists and surgeons.

The major advantage of SD plasma over FFP and the other PI plasmas is the extreme safety with regard to transfusion-related acute lung injury (TRALI), which is a leading cause of transfusion-induced death in industrialized countries.[11,29] After transfusion of >6.5 million units, only one case of TRALI (minor morbidity, grade 2), possibly caused by SD plasma, was reported from France[70] after transfusion of >700,000 units of SD plasma between 2003 and 2008.[29] [This was later regarded as not attributable to the plasma transfusion (G. Andreu, personal communication).] After transfusion of a somewhat higher number of quarantine plasma units in the same period, the hemovigilance data from France indicate a frequency of TRALI of 1 in 25,000 units.[29] The dubious minor morbidity TRALI case observed in France was with SD plasma prepared from a pool of only 60 L (100 apheresis units of 600 mL), whereas after transfusion of plasma prepared from 380-L pools (from 630 apheresis units to 1520 recovered FFP units), no cases have been documented where the cause could be traced to SD plasma (this includes >350,000 units transfused in the United Kingdom after introduction of its Serious Hazards of Transfusion hemovigilance system in 1996).

Another advantage of SD plasma over FFP is its markedly lower rate of allergic reactions (see Chapters 7 and 8).[62,64] This was supported by the 2006 Austrian hemovigilance register data, which report 14 allergic reactions after 23,500 units of FFP, and 2 after 52,400 units of Octaplas ($p < 0.0001$; W. R. Mayr, Medical University of Vienna, Austria, personal communication). Allergic reaction rates also declined dramatically and significantly after switching from standard FFP to Octaplas in Finland (T. Krusius, Finnish Red Cross Blood Service, personal communication).

The advantages of SD plasma with respect to TRALI are best explained by the dilution effect of pooling and the possible neutralization of antibodies by residual leukocytes or soluble antigens in the plasma units. The lower number of allergic reactions is likely the result of the dilution effect on antibodies and allergens. Also not to be excluded is a possible effect of SD treatment on activated lipids involved in TRALI.

Methylene Blue/Light-Treated Plasma

Little clinical research has focused on the efficacy and tolerance of MB plasma, despite the fact that it is in widespread clinical use (Table 5-3). One recent prospective cohort study in 90 patients with thrombotic thrombocytopenic purpura (TTP)[79] confirmed the findings of one small observational study[75] and one retrospective analysis,[76] which suggested lower remission and higher relapse rates under plasma exchange with MB plasma when compared with standard FFP. The reason for the observed inferior efficacy of MB plasma in TTP remains to be explained, particularly in view of the fact that vWF-cleaving protease (ADAMTS-13) activity, which must be replaced efficiently in TTP patients, seems to be just as well preserved in MB plasma as in all other plasma types.[32,34,80-84] Two retrospective analyses found an increased demand for plasma and plasma derivatives after switching from FFP to MB plasma,[72,74] though others could not confirm these findings.[11,77] A serious allergic adverse event resulting in patient death has been reported after transfusion of MB plasma,[70] but no increase of allergic reactions in general has been documented after transfusion of MB plasma.

Psoralen/Ultraviolet Light-Treated Plasma (Intercept Plasma)

Four studies have examined the efficacy and tolerance of Intercept plasma in healthy volunteers and in patients with congenital coagulation factor deficiencies, TTP, and coagulopathy in liver diseases (Table 5-4). A crossover trial of healthy volunteers treated with warfarin demonstrated equal correction of prothrombin time (PT) and equivalent increases in Factor VII plasma levels after transfusion of autologous Intercept plasma and autologous FFP, respectively.[85]

Table 5-3. Clinical Trials of Methylene Blue/Light-Treated Plasma

Study Group	Design	Clinical Setting	Main Results
Wieding, Neumeyer (1992)[71]	Observational: MB plasma (n = 103)	Complex coagulopathy	No specific adverse events
Hernandez et al (1999)[72]	Retrospective analysis: 5912 units of MB plasma	All indications	0.6% adverse reactions Plasma demand increased by 20% after switching from FFP to MB plasma
Simonsen, Sorensen (1999)[73]	Prospective, randomized crossover: 12 healthy volunteers, autologous MB plasma vs autologous FFP	Phase I study	No adverse events after autologous MB plasma or autologous FFP
Wieding et al (1999)[53]	Prospective, randomized (n = 71): SD plasma vs MB plasma	Cardiopulmonary bypass surgery	No clinical difference No increase in protein S and plasmin inhibitor levels after SD plasma
Atance et al (2001)[74]	Retrospective analysis: three 1-year periods (n = 2967)	All indications	Demand of plasma and cryoprecipitate increased by 56% and 50%, respectively, after switching from FFP to MB plasma
de la Rubia et al (2001)[75]	Observational: MB plasma (n = 7) vs FFP (n = 13)	TTP, plasma exchange	Remission rate: 57% vs 69% (ns) Number of plasma exchanges greater and duration of hospitalization significantly longer in the MB plasma group

(Continued)

Table 5-3. Clinical Trials of Methylene Blue/Light-Treated Plasma (Continued)

Study Group	Design	Clinical Setting	Main Results
Alvarez-Larrán et al (2004)[76]	Retrospective analysis: 43 patients, 27 treatment episodes with MB plasma and 29 with FFP	TTP, plasma exchange	Higher mortality and recurrence rate with MB plasma
Cid et al (2005)[77]	Retrospective analysis: seven 1-year periods, more than 200,000 MB plasma units transfused	All indications	No increase in MB plasma/red cell ratios after switching to MB plasma
Politis et al (2007)[78]	Retrospective analysis: 5 years, 8500 units of MB plasma and 54,435 units of FFP	All indications	Adverse reactions: 1:8500 with MB plasma and 1:2177 with FFP (ns)
del Rio-Garma et al (2008)[79]	Prospective cohort: 90 patients, 63 treatment episodes with MB plasma and 39 with FFP	TTP, plasma exchange	MB plasma required more exchanges and larger plasma volumes Lower remission and higher relapse rates with MB plasma

MB = methylene blue; FFP = Fresh Frozen Plasma; SD = solvent/detergent; ns = not significant; TTP = thrombotic thrombocytopenic purpura.

Table 5-4. Clinical Trials of Amotosalen/Ultraviolet-Light-Treated Plasma (Intercept* Plasma)

Study Group	Design	Clinical Setting	Main Results
Hambleton et al (2002)[85]	Prospective crossover: 27 healthy volunteers, autologous Intercept plasma vs autologous FFP, retransfusion after anticoagulation with warfarin	Phase I study	No difference in PT and Factor VII kinetics
de Alarcon et al (2005)[38]	Observational (n = 34): kinetics of fibrinogen; Factors II, V, VII, X, XI, and XIII; and protein C	Congenital coagulation factor deficiencies	Correction of aPTT or PT Effective hemostasis in 13 patients with bleeding or invasive procedures
Mintz et al (2006)[86]	Prospective, randomized, controlled Phase III: Intercept plasma (n = 17) vs FFP (n = 18)	TTP, plasma exchange	Equal remission rates
Mintz et al (2006)[87]	Prospective, randomized, controlled: Intercept plasma (n = 60) vs FFP (n = 61)	Coagulopathy in liver disease	No difference in PT correction Equal clinical hemostasis

*Cerus Corp, Concord, CA.
FFP = fresh frozen plasma; PT = prothrombin time; aPTT = activated partial thromboplastin time; TTP = thrombotic thrombocytopenic purpura.

Factor VII posttransfusion half-life times did not differ significantly between the two plasma types. De Alcaron et al examined 34 patients with hereditary coagulation factor or inhibitor deficiencies (fibrinogen; Factors II, V, VII, X, and XI; or protein C).[38] Intercept plasma was transfused for kinetic studies and for treatment or prophylaxis of bleeding. Kinetics and therapeutic efficacy were consistent with standard FFP, except for shorter fibrinogen, Factor II, and Factor XIII half-life times. A striking finding was that 60% of the patients experienced urticaria. One randomized controlled trial of plasma exchange in TTP observed no differences in clinical efficacy or tolerance between Intercept plasma and FFP.[86] Another prospective, controlled, double-blinded, randomized study determined the efficacy and safety of Intercept plasma compared with conventional FFP in 121 patients with acquired coagulopathy accompanying liver disease, among them 51 patients receiving liver transplants.[87] No differences with regard to clinical hemostasis and correction of PT were observed between groups.

Riboflavin/Light-Treated Plasma (Mirasol Plasma)

CE status was granted for Mirasol plasma in 2008 based on protein quality data reported, along with a toxicology dossier and human clinical safety data on products infused into patients. Subsequently, observational clinical studies have been undertaken at several sites in Europe to assess product performance in routine use, but the results of this work are not yet published (A. Ettinger, CaridianBCT, personal communication).

Cost-Effectiveness

Because of the very low residual risk for recognized viral infections, the cost-effectiveness of PI is rather low in industrialized countries when compared to other strategies to reduce noninfectious transfusion risks[88] but is comparable to the cost-effectiveness of nucleic acid testing of blood products. When only the benefit of viral inactivation is considered, the cost of a quality-adjusted life year has been calculated to approach US$10 million for SD plasma, and this cost may be presumed to be similar for PI of plasma by other methods and for quarantine plasma (see Chapter 7).[11] During early stages of emerging infections[89] and in resource-limited countries with high residual infection risk, the cost-effectiveness is likely much better, but no calculations have been published thus far.[29] When the benefit accrued from the reduced incidence of TRALI is taken into consideration, the cost per life year saved for pooled SD-treated plasma is reduced to between US$40,000 and 170,000, depending on patient age.[90] Further reductions can be obtained when the reduction in allergic/anaphylactic adverse events and advantage of universal ABO-independent SD plasma are taken into account.[28] In countries where all plasma supplies must be either pathogen inactivated or quarantined, concerns about cost-effectiveness take second place to legal considerations.[29] The cost-effectiveness of minipool SD-treated plasma has not yet been calculated but should be favorable in resource-limited countries with high infection risks.

Pathogen Inactivation of Cryoprecipitate

Solvent/Detergent Treatment

Cryoprecipitates prepared from Octaplas were found to have reduced levels of vWF and also lacked the highest multimers of vWF but had adequate levels of fibrinogen.[91] Throughout most of the 1990s Octaplas also lacked the highest multimers of vWF. However, optimization of the manufacturing process and introduction of new filters has since changed the vWF multimeric profile of Octaplas to normal (T-E. Svae, Octapharma, personal communication).[92] The authors are not aware of any studies involving preparation of cryoprecipitate from Octaplas with a normal vWF multimer profile.

Octapharma AG has produced an SD-treated cryoprecipitate for Norway since 1992. The product is produced by SD treatment of cryoprecipitate from reconstituted plasma, with further processing equivalent to other single inactivated Factor VIII/vWF products without further purification. After dispersal into 10-mL vials, the product is lyophilized. The vial content ranges from 250 to 500 IU vWF antigen with a normal vWF multimer profile and 300 to 600 mg fibrinogen. The cryoprecipitate is most commonly used to treat patients with congenital fibrinogen deficiency, but it has also been used successfully to treat bleeding in vWF-deficient patients. The mean consumption has been 100 to 200 vials per year, which indicates the minor importance of this product.

Particularly suited for use in blood banks in resource-limited countries is SD treatment of minipool cryoprecipitate in a single-use bag system.[93] The method showed >93% mean recovery of Factor VIII coagulant activity, vWF ristocetin cofactor, and clottable fibrinogen. A PI cryoprecipitate depleted of isoagglutinins and enriched in functional Factor VIII, vWF, and clottable fibrinogen represents a further improvement of the minipool method.[94]

Methylene Blue/Light Treatment

MB/light-treated cryoprecipitate has been produced from MB plasma in the United Kingdom (see Chapter 10).[95-97] The reduction of fibrinogen in MB plasma is reflected in the cryoprecipitate. The fibrinogen content can be somewhat increased by modifying storage conditions; however, this decreases the Factor VIII content.[97]

In spite of UK clinical use of MB cryoprecipitate, the authors are not aware of reports published on its efficacy.

Amotosalen/Ultraviolet Light-Treated Cryoprecipitate (Intercept Cryoprecipitate)

Production of cryoprecipitate from Intercept plasma has been reported (see Chapter 10).[98] The product has not been in clinical use, however (M. Witzöe, Cerus, personal communication).

Conclusion

More than 6.5 million units of the biopharmaceutical SD-treated pooled plasma units (Octaplas) have been transfused since 1992. The product is licensed in 29 countries worldwide and is currently expected to be replaced by the newly licensed prion-reduced product OctaplasLG. Of the single-unit inactivated plasmas, >4 million units of MB-treated plasma have been transfused in Europe since the 1990s, and one method (Macopharma) has gained CE status for

Table 5-5. Properties of Different Types of Therapeutic Plasma

Therapeutic Plasma Type	PI	Free of Cells and Cell Fragments	Risk of TRALI Abolished	Allergic Reactions Reduced	Standardized Coagulation Factor Potencies	Full Clinical Efficacy in All Settings
SD plasma	Yes	Yes	Yes*	Yes	Yes	Yes
MB plasma	Yes	No	No	No	No	No†
Intercept plasma	Yes	No	No	No	No	Yes
Mirasol plasma	Yes	No	No	No	No	?‡
Standard FFP	No	No	No	No	No	Yes

*One dubious case of TRALI (minor morbidity: grade 2) after transfusion of SD plasma from 60-L pool (dilution: 1:100); no cases after transfusion of >6.5 million units of SD from 380-L pools (dilution: 1:630 to 1:1520).

†Reduced efficacy in plasma exchange in thrombotic thrombocytopenic purpura.

‡So far only clinical studies for the granting of Conformité Européenne (CE) status.

PI = pathogen inactivation; TRALI = transfusion-related acute lung injury; SD = solvent/detergent; MB = methylene blue; FFP = fresh frozen plasma.

application in blood banks. Less experience has been gained with amotosalen-treated plasma (Intercept plasma) or riboflavin-treated plasma (Mirasol plasma), which were granted CE marks in 2006 and 2008, respectively. None of the PI products currently licensed or CE marked in Europe are licensed in the United States. No toxic or immunologic adverse reactions have so far been observed for these products. Except for TTP treatment with MB plasma, clinical efficacy of the PI products seems to be similar to that of FFP. The European SD-treated pooled plasma has a very high safety profile with regard to TRALI and causes significantly fewer allergic transfusion reactions than FFP. The properties of the PI products are summarized in Table 5-5. Adverse reactions of PI plasma are now closely monitored by national hemovigilance systems. A minipool method for SD treatment of plasma/cryoprecipitate has been developed for use in blood banks in resource-limited countries.

References

1. Burnouf-Radosevich M, Burnouf T, Huart JJ. A pasteurized therapeutic plasma. Infusionsther Transfusionsmed 1992;19:91-4.
2. Burnouf T, Radosevich M, El-Ekiaby M, et al. Nanofiltration of single plasma donations: Feasibility study. Vox Sang 2003;84:111-19.
3. Prince AM, Horowitz B, Brotman B. Sterilization of hepatitis and HTLV-III viruses by exposure to tri(n-butyl)phosphate and sodium cholate. Lancet 1986; i:706-10.
4. Biesert L, Shartono H. Solvent/detergent treatment of human plasma—a very robust method for virus inactivation. Validation of virus safety of Octaplas. Vox Sang 1998;74(Suppl 1):207-12.
5. Horowitz B, Bonomo R, Prince AM, et al. Solvent/detergent-treated plasma. A virus-inactivated substitute for fresh frozen plasma. Blood 1992;79:826-33.
6. Hellstern P, Sachse H, Schwinn H, Oberfrank K. Manufacture and in-vitro characterization of a solvent/detergent-treated plasma. Vox Sang 1992;63:178-85.
7. Pelletier JPR, Transue S, Snyder EL. Pathogen inactivation techniques. Best Pract Res Clin Haematol 2006;19:205-42.
8. Roberts P. Resistance of vaccinia virus to inactivation by solvent/detergent treatment of blood products. Biologicals 2000;28:29-32.
9. Solheim BG, Rollag H, Svennevig JL, et al. Viral safety of solvent/detergent-treated plasma. Transfusion 2000;40:84-90.
10. Rollag H, Solheim BG, Svennevig JL. Viral safety of blood derivatives by immune neutralization. Vox Sang 1998;74(Suppl 1):213-17.

11. Solheim BG, Cid J, Osselaer JC. Pathogen reduction technologies. In: Lozano M, Contreras M, Blajchman M, eds. Global perspectives in transfusion medicine. Bethesda, MD: AABB Press, 2006:103-48.
12. Neisser-Svae A, Bailey A, Gregori L, et al. Prion removal effect of a specific affinity ligand introduced in the manufacturing process of the pharmaceutical quality solvent/detergent (S/D)-treated plasma OctaplasLG. Vox Sang 2009;97:226-33.
13. Svae TE, Neisser-Svae A, Bailey A, et al. Prion safety of transfusion plasma and plasma-derivatives typically used for prophylactic treatment. Transfus Apher Sci 2008;39:59-67.
14. Solheim BG. Universal pathogen-reduced plasma in elective open-heart surgery and liver resection. Review. Clin Med Res 2006;4:209-17.
15. Tollofsrud S, Noddeland H, Svennevig JL, et al. Universal fresh frozen plasma (Uniplas): A safe product in open-heart surgery. Intensive Care Med 2003;29: 1736-43.
16. Solheim BG, Granov DA, Juralev VA, et al. Universal fresh-frozen plasma (Uniplas): An exploratory study in adult patients undergoing elective liver resection. Vox Sang 2005;89:19-26.
17. Burnouf T, Goubran HA, Radosevich M, et al. A process for solvent/detergent treatment of plasma for transfusion at blood centers that use a disposable-bag system. Transfusion 2006;46:2100-8.
18. El-Ekiaby M, Radosevich M, Goubran H, et al. New methods of plasma fractionation—a presentation of the "mini-pool" fractionation procedure developed in Egypt. ISBT Science Series 2009;4:99-106.
19. Burnouf T, Goubran HA, Radosevich M, et al. Impact of Triton X-100 on alpha$_2$-antiplasmin (SERPINF2) activity in solvent/detergent treated plasma. Biologicals 2007;35:349-53.
20. Clifton CE. Photodynamic action of certain dyes on the inactivation of staphylococcus bacteriophage. Proc Soc Exp Biol Med 1931;28:745-6.
21. Wagner SJ. Virus inactivation in blood components by photoactive phenothiazine dyes. Transfus Med Rev 2002;16:61-6.
22. Lambrecht B, Mohr H, Knüver-Hopf J, Schmitt H. Photoinactivation of viruses in human fresh plasma by phenothiazine dyes in combination with visible light. Vox Sang 1991;60:207-13.
23. Mohr H, Lambrecht B, Seltz A. Photodynamic virus inactivation of blood components. Immunol Invest 1995;24:73-85.
24. Ciravino V, McCullough T, Cimino G, Sullivan T. Preclinical safety profile of plasma prepared using the INTERCEPT blood system. Vox Sang 2003;85: 171-82.
25. Goodrich RP, Edrich RA, Li J, Seghatchian J. The Mirasol system for pathogen reduction of platelets and plasma: An overview of current status and future trends. Transfus Apher Sci 2006;35:5-17.
26. Solheim BG, Seghatchian J. Pathogen inactivation. In: Simon TL, Snyder EL, Solheim BG, et al, eds. Rossi's principles of transfusion medicine. Bethesda, MD: AABB Press, 2009:801-10.
27. Kumar V, Lockerbie O, Keil SD, et al. Riboflavin and UV-light based pathogen reduction: Extent and consequence of DNA damage at the molecular level. Photochem Photobiol 2004;80:15-21.

28. Solheim BG, Seghatchian J. Update on pathogen reduction technology for therapeutic plasma: An overview. Transfus Apher Sci 2006;35:83-90.
29. Prowse C. Properties of pathogen-inactivated plasma components. Transfus Med Rev 2009;23:124-33.
30. Ciaravi V, McCullough T, Dayan AD. Pharmacokinetic and toxicology assessment of INTERCEPT (S-59 and UVA treated) platelets. Human Exp Toxicol 2001;20:533-50.
31. Beeck H, Hellstern P. In vitro characterization of solvent/detergent-treated human plasma and of quarantine fresh frozen plasma. Vox Sang 1998;74 (Suppl 1):219-23.
32. Heger A, Svae T-E, Neisser-Svae A, et al. Biochemical quality of the pharmaceutical licensed plasma OctaplasLG after implementation of a novel prion protein (PrPSc) removal technology and reduction of the solvent/detergent (S/D) process time. Vox Sang 2009;97:219-25.
33. Aznar JA, Molina R, Montoro JM. Factor VIII/von Willebrand complex in methylene blue-treated plasma. Transfusion 1999;39:748-50.
34. Osselaer JC, Debry C, Goffaux M, et al. Coagulation function in fresh-frozen plasma prepared with two photochemical treatment methods: Methylene blue and amotosalen. Transfusion 2008;48:108-17.
35. Pock K, Heger A, Janisch S, et al. Thrombin generation capacity is impaired in methylene-blue treated plasma compared to normal levels in single-donor fresh-frozen plasma, a licensed solvent/detergent-treated plasma (Octaplas) and a development product (Uniplas). Transfus Apher Sci 2007;37:223-31.
36. Depasse F, Sensebe L, Seghatchian J, et al. The influence of methylene blue light treatment and methylene blue removal filter on fibrinogen activity states and fibrin polymerization indices. Transfus Apher Sci 2005;33:63-9.
37. Cardigan R, Philpot K, Cookson P, Luddington R. Thrombin generation in methylene blue-treated plasma and cryoprecipitate. Transfusion 2009;49: 696-703.
38. de Alarcon P, Benjamin R, Dugdale M, et al. Fresh frozen plasma prepared with amotosalen (S-59) photochemical pathogen inactivation: Transfusion of patients with congenital coagulation factor deficiencies. Transfusion 2005; 45:1362-72.
39. Singh Y, Sawyer LS, Pinkoski LS, et al. Photochemical treatment of plasma with amotosalen and long-wavelength light inactivates pathogens while retaining coagulation function. Transfusion 2006;46:1168-77.
40. Hornsey VS, Drummond O, Morrison A, et al. Pathogen reduction of fresh plasma using riboflavin and ultraviolet light: Effects on plasma coagulation proteins. Transfusion 2009;49:2167-72.
41. Runkel S, Haubelt H, Hitzler W, Hellstern P. The quality of plasma collected by automated apheresis and of recovered plasma from leukodepleted whole blood. Transfusion 2005;45:427-32.
42. Hellstern P. Solvent/detergent-treated plasma: Composition, efficacy, and safety. Curr Opin Hematol 2004;11:346-50.
43. Solheim BG, Hellstern P. Composition, efficacy, and safety of S/D-treated plasma. Transfusion 2003;43:1176-8.

44. Heiden M, Salge U, Breitner-Ruddock S, et al. Significant differences between S/D plasma qualities of different origin (abstract). Transfusion 2003; 43(Suppl):56A.
45. Salge-Bartels U, Breitner-Ruddock S, Hunfeld A, et al. Are quality differences responsible for different adverse reactions reported for SD-plasma for USA and Europe? Transfus Med 2006;16:266-75.
46. Cid J, Ramiro L, Martinez N, et al. Quantitative and qualitative analysis of proteins in fresh frozen plasma obtained from whole blood donations and prepared with two photochemical treatments. Transfus Apher Sci 2008;39: 114-21.
47. Bihm DJ, Ettinger A, Buytaert-Hoefen KA, et al. Characterization of plasma protein activity in riboflavin and UV light-treated fresh frozen plasma during 2 years of storage at –30 C. Vox Sang 2010;98:108-15.
48. Hellstern P, Larbig E, Walz GA, et al. Prospective study on efficacy and tolerability of solvent/detergent-treated plasma in intensive care unit patients. Infusther Transfusmed 1993;20(Suppl 2):16-18.
49. Inbal A, Epstein O, Blickstein D, et al. Evaluation of solvent/detergent treated plasma in the management of patients with hereditary and acquired coagulation disorders. Blood Coagul Fibrinolysis 1993;4:599-604.
50. Solheim BG, Svennevig JL, Mohr B, et al. The use of Octaplas in patients undergoing open heart surgery. In: Müller-Berghaus G, ed. DIC: Pathogenesis, diagnosis and therapy of disseminated intravascular fibrin formation. Amsterdam: Elsevier, 1993:253-62.
51. Baudoux E, Margraff U, Coenen A, et al. Hemovigilance: Clinical tolerance of solvent-detergent treated plasma. Vox Sang 1998;74(Suppl 1):237-9.
52. Horowitz MS, Pehta JC. SD plasma in TTP and coagulation factor deficiencies for which no concentrates are available. Vox Sang 1998;74(Suppl 1): 231-5.
53. Wieding JU, Rathgeber J, Zenker D, et al. Prospective, randomized, and controlled study on solvent/detergent versus methylene blue/light virus-inactivated plasma. Transfusion 1999;39(Suppl 10):23.
54. Williamson IM, Llewelyn CA, Fisher NC, et al. A randomized trial of solvent/ detergent-treated and standard fresh-frozen plasma in the coagulopathy of liver disease and liver transplantation. Transfusion 1999;39:1227-34.
55. Beck KH, Mortelmans Y, Kretschmer V, et al. Comparison of solvent/detergent-inactivated plasma and fresh frozen plasma under routine clinical conditions. Infusther Transfusmed 2000;27:144-8.
56. Lerner RG, Nelson J, Scorcia E, et al. Evaluation of solvent/detergent-treated plasma in patients with a prolonged prothrombin time. Vox Sang 2000;79: 161-7.
57. Haubelt H, Blome M, Kiessling AH, et al. Effects of solvent/detergent-treated plasma and fresh frozen plasma on hemostasis and fibrinolysis in complex coagulopathy following open-heart surgery. Vox Sang 2002;82:9-14.
58. de Jonge J, Groenland THN, Metselaar HJ, et al. Fibrinolysis during liver transplantation is enhanced by using solvent/detergent virus-inactivated plasma (ESDEP). Anesth Analg 2002;94:1127-31.

59. de Jonge J, Groenland THN, Metselaar HJ, et al. Liver transplantation, solvent/detergent treated plasma and antifibrinolytics. Anesth Analg 2003;96: 1230-1.
60. Solheim BG, Bergan A, Brosstad F, et al. Fibrinolysis during liver transplant and use of solvent/detergent virus-inactivated plasma (ESDEP/Octaplas). Anesth Analg 2003;96:1230-1.
61. Chekrizova V, Murphy WG. Solvent-detergent plasma: Use in neonatal patients, in adult and pediatric patients with liver disease and in obstetric and gynaecological emergencies. Transfus Med 2006;16:85-91.
62. McCarthy LJ. The experience of treating patients with thrombotic thrombocytopenic purpura with solvent detergent plasma. Br J Haematol 2006;133: 107.
63. Santagostino E, Mancuso ME, Morfini M, et al. Solvent/detergent plasma for prevention of bleeding in recessively inherited coagulation disorders: Dosing, pharmacokinetics and clinical efficacy. Haematologica 2006;91:634-9.
64. Scully M, Longair I, Flynn M, et al. Cryosupernatant and solvent detergent fresh-frozen plasma (Octaplas) usage in a single centre in acute thrombotic thrombocytopenic purpura. Vox Sang 2007;93:154-8.
65. Leebeek FWG, Schipperus MR, van Vliet HHDM. Coagulation factor levels in solvent/detergent-treated plasma. Transfusion 1999;39:1150-1.
66. Mast AE, Stadanlick JE, Lockett JM, Dietzen DJ. Solvent/detergent-treated plasma has decreased antitrypsin activity and absent antiplasmin activity. Blood 1999;94:3922-7.
67. Flamholz R, Jeon HR, Baron JM, Baron BW. Study of three patients with thrombotic thrombocytopenic purpura exchanged with solvent/detergent-treated plasma: Is its decreased protein S activity clinically related to their development of deep vein thromboses? J Clin Apher 2000;15:169-72.
68. Yarranton H, Cohen H, Pavord SR, et al. Venous thromboembolism associated with the management of acute thrombotic thrombocytopenic purpura. Br J Haematol 2003;121:778-85.
69. Hellstern P. Fresh-frozen plasma, pathogen-reduced single-donor plasma or bio-pharmaceutical plasma? Transfus Apher Sci 2008;39:69-74.
70. Agence Française de sécurité sanitaire des produits de santé. Rapport annuel hémovigilance 2008. Saint Denis, France: AFSSAPS, 2009.
71. Wieding JU, Neumeyer H. Initial experience with methylene blue virus inactivated fresh frozen plasma: Results of a clinical and in vitro study. Infusionsther Transfusionsmed 1992;19:84-90.
72. Hernandez JM, Castella D, Claparols M, et al. Clinical use of fresh frozen plasma virus inactivated with methylene blue (abstract). Transfusion 1999;39 (Suppl 1):25S.
73. Simonsen AC, Sorensen H. Clinical tolerance of methylene blue virus-inactivated plasma: A randomized cross-over trial in 12 healthy human volunteers. Vox Sang 1999;77:210-17.
74. Atance R, Pereira A, Ramírez B. Transfusing methylene blue-photoinactivated plasma instead of FFP is associated with an increased demand for plasma and cryoprecitpitate. Transfusion 2001;41:1548-52.

75. de la Rubia J, Arriag F, Linares D, et al. Role of methylene blue-treated fresh frozen plasma in the response to plasma exchange in patients with thrombotic thrombocytopenic purpura. Br J Haematol 2001;114:721-3.
76. Alvarez-Larrán A, del Rio J, Ramirez C, et al. Methylene blue-photoinactivated plasma vs. fresh-frozen plasma as replacement fluid for plasma exchange in thrombotic thrombocytopenic purpura. Vox Sang 2004;86:246-51.
77. Cid J, Puig L, Pla RP, Hernandez JM. (Over) use of methylene blue-treated fresh frozen plasma? 7-years experience (abstract). Transfusion 2005;45 (Suppl 3):74A.
78. Politis C, Kavallierou L, Hantziara S, et al. Quality and safety of fresh-frozen plasma inactivated and leucoreduced with the Theraflex methylene blue system including the Blueflex filter: 5 years´ experience. Vox Sang 2007;92: 319-26.
79. del Rio-Garma J, Alvarez-Larrán A, Martínez C, et al. Methylene blue-photoinactivated plasma versus quarantine fresh frozen plasma in thrombotic thrombocytopenic purpura: A multicentric, prospective trial. Br J Haematol 2008;143:39-45.
80. Furlan M, Robles R, Galbusera M, et al. Von Willebrand factor-cleaving protease in thrombotic thrombocytopenic purpura and the hemolytic-uremic syndrome. N Engl J Med 1998;339:1578-84.
81. Cardigan R, Allford S, Williamson L. Levels of von Willebrand factor-cleaving protease are normal in methylene blue-treated fresh-frozen plasma. Br J Haematol 2002;117:253-4.
82. Yarranton H, Lawrie AS, Purdy G, et al. Comparison of von Willebrand factor antigen, von Willebrand factor-cleaving protease and protein S in blood components used for treatment of thrombotic thrombocytopenic purpura. Transfus Med 2004;14:39-44.
83. Fontana S, Kremer-Hovinga JA, Studt JD, et al. Plasma therapy in thrombotic thrombocytopenic purpura: Review of the literature and the Bern experience in a subgroup of patients with severe acquired ADAMTS-13 deficiency. Semin Hematol 2004;41:48-59.
84. del Rio-Garma J, Pereira A, Arroyo JL, et al. ADAMTS-13 activity and von Willebrand factor levels in methylene blue photo-inactivated plasma processed by either the Springe method or an "in house" system. Vox Sang 2008; 95:101-5.
85. Hambleton J, Wages D, Radu-Radulescu L, et al. Pharmacokinetic study of FFP photochemically treated with amotosalen (S-59) and UV light compared to FFP in healthy volunteers anticoagulated with warfarin. Transfusion 2002; 42:1302-7.
86. Mintz PD, Neff A, MacKenzie M, et al. A randomized, controlled phase III trial of therapeutic plasma exchange with fresh-frozen plasma (FFP) prepared with amotosalen and ultraviolet A light compared to untreated FFP in thrombotic thrombocytopenic purpura. Transfusion 2006;46:1693-704.
87. Mintz PD, Bass NM, Petz LD, et al. Photochemically treated fresh frozen plasma for transfusion of patients with acquired coagulopathy of liver disease. Blood 2006;107:3753-60.

88. Klein HG. Pathogen inactivation technology: Cleansing the blood supply. J Intern Med 2005;257:224-37.
89. Rasonglès P, Isola H, Kientz D, et al. Rapid implementation of photochemical pathogen inactivation (INTERCEPT) for preparation of platelet components during an epidemic of chikungunya virus (abstract). Vox Sang 2006; 91(Suppl 3):32.
90. Riedler GF, Haycox AR, Duggan AK, Dakin HA. Cost-effectiveness of solvent/detergent-treated fresh-frozen plasma. Vox Sang 2003;85:88-95.
91. Keeling DM, Luddington R, Allain JP, et al. Cryoprecipitate prepared from plasma virally inactivated by the solvent detergent method. Br J Haematol 1997;96:194-7.
92. Heger A, Kannicht C, Römisch J, Svae T-E. Normal levels of ADAMS13 and factor H are present in the pharmaceutically licensed plasma for transfusion (Octaplas) and in the universally applicable plasma (Uniplas) in development. Vox Sang 2007;92:206-12.
93. Burnouf T, Goubran HA, Radosevich M, et al. A minipool process for solvent-detergent treatment of cryoprecipitate at blood centres using a disposable bag system. Vox Sang 2006;91:56-62.
94. Burnouf T, Caron C, Radosevich M, et al. Properties of a concentrated minipool solvent-detergent treated cryoprecipitate processed in single-use bag systems. Haemophilia 2008;14:956-62.
95. Hornsey VS, Krailadsiri P, MacDonald S, et al. Coagulation factor content of cryoprecipitate prepared from methylene blue plus light virus-inactivated plasma. Br J Haematol 2000;109:665-70.
96. Aznar JA, Bonanad S, Montoro JM, et al. Influence of methylene blue photoinactivation treatment on coagulation factors from fresh frozen plasma, cryoprecipitates and cryosupernatants. Vox Sang 2000;79:156-60.
97. Hornsey VS, Young DA, Docherty A, et al. Cryoprecipitate prepared from plasma treated with methylene blue plus light: Increasing the fibrinogen concentration. Transfus Med 2004;14:369-74.
98. Wages D, Eden P, Smyders J, et al. Preparation of cryoprecipitate from photochemically treated fresh frozen plasma (abstract). Transfusion 2000;40(Suppl): 63S.

In: AuBuchon JP, Prowse CV, eds.
Pathogen Inactivation: The Penultimate Paradigm Shift
Bethesda, MD: AABB Press, 2010

6

Pathogen Inactivation of Platelets

JEFFREY McCULLOUGH, MD

SEVERAL PATHOGEN INACTIVATION (PI) TECHNIques have been investigated for application to platelets in an attempt to improve the safety of this component. This chapter describes the results of structured clinical trials of the two of these platelet products that are furthest along in development and are being implemented in clinical practice.

The application of amotosalen and ultraviolet (UV) light has been developed by the Cerus Corporation (Concord, CA) as the Intercept system. After apheresis collection of platelets or their production from whole blood units, the photosensitizing compound amo-

---

Jeffrey McCullough, MD, Director, Institute for Engineering in Medicine, and Professor of Laboratory Medicine, University of Minnesota Medical School, Minneapolis, Minnesota

The author has disclosed no conflicts of interest.

tosalen is mixed with the unit's contents while flowing into an illumination bag. The unit is exposed to UVA light for several minutes before being transferred to a bag containing a compound adsorption device (CAD) that removes unreacted amotosalen and reaction byproducts. Finally, the unit is transferred to a storage bag for subsequent transfusion.

The use of riboflavin as a photosensitizer has been developed by CaridianBCT (Lakewood, CO) as the Mirasol system. This method is similar to Intercept except for the spectrum of UV light used (UVA + UVB) and the lack of application of a device to remove the riboflavin or its byproducts because these are considered naturally occurring compounds.

In-Vivo Phase I and II Studies

Amotosalen

The first reported experience with platelets subjected to PI using the amotosalen method involved determination of the posttransfusion recovery and lifespan of radiolabeled platelets in normal research subjects.[1] Autologous platelet concentrates containing approximately 3×10^{11} platelets in approximately 250 mL of plasma were collected by apheresis using the CS3000 blood cell separator (Fenwal Inc, Lake Zurich, IL). The platelets were treated with amotosalen and UV light.[2,3] Following pathogen inactivation, the platelet concentrates were stored for 5 days at 20 to 24 C with continuous agitation, and on day 5 a 10-mL aliquot of platelets was labeled with ^{111}Indium and injected into the subjects. There was a slight but statistically significant reduction in posttransfusion recovery and lifespan compared to similar but untreated platelets (Table 6-1). Following this Phase I study, amotosalen-treated platelets were given in a Phase II study to 13 thrombocytopenic patients.[4,5] The 1-hour posttransfusion platelet count increment and the corrected count increment (which takes into account platelet dose and the size of the patient) were both statistically significantly less than the control, non-pathogen-inactivated platelets (Table 6-2). After transfusion, the bleeding time decreased from 28.7 ±2.5 to 14.3 ±6.5 minutes in control patients and from 29.2 ±1.6 to 19.3 ±9.5 minutes in those receiving the PI platelets (Table 6-2). The extent of the

Table 6-1. Posttransfusion Recovery and Lifespan of Platelets Subjected to Pathogen Inactivation*

	Amosotalen†			Riboflavin‡		
	n	% Recovery	Lifespan (days)	n	% Recovery	Lifespan (hours)
Control	16	50.3 ±7.7	6.0 ±1.2	29	66.5 ±13.4	142 ±26
Pathogen inactivation	16	42.5 ±8.7*	4.8 ±1.3*	29	50 ±18.9§	104 ±26§

*$p < 0.01$.
†From Snyder et al.[1]
‡From AuBuchon et al.
§$p < 0.05$.

decrease (improvement) in bleeding time after transfusion of PI platelets was not statistically significantly different from control platelets (Table 6-2), although the decrease with the PI platelets was not as extensive as that accomplished with control platelets. In another section of this study, similar posttransfusion recovery and lifespan studies were performed on PI platelets subjected to gamma irradiation, routinely used to prevent graft-vs-host disease. The addition of gamma irradiation did not further reduce the posttransfusion recovery or lifespan of the amotosalen PI platelets.

Riboflavin

PI is also performed using riboflavin as the photoinactivator.[6,7] In the first Phase I study of the in-vivo results of riboflavin-treated platelets, AuBuchon et al[8] collected platelets by apheresis from 29 normal subjects each on two occasions. In random order, one collection was studied without further treatment, and the other collection was subjected to PI using the riboflavin technology and then studied. Platelets were stored for 5 days, radiolabeled with ^{111}Indium oxine, and injected into the subjects. The percent recovery in the control subjects was 66.5 ±13.4 compared to 50.0 ±18.9 ($p < 0.05$) in the subjects who received the PI platelets (Table 6-1). The survival of transfused platelets was 142 ±26 hours in patients who received the untreated control platelets and 104 ±26 hours in patients who received the PI platelets (Table 6-1). This reduction in lifespan of riboflavin-treated platelets was also statistically significant ($p < 0.05$). Thus, these studies were similar to those with the amotosalen-treated platelets in showing that the recovery and survival of PI platelets are decreased compared to untreated platelets.

Phase III Clinical Trials of Pathogen-Inactivated Platelets

EuroSPRITE

The first reported large-scale clinical trial of PI platelets was a prospectively randomized controlled trial of amotosalen-treated PI buffy-coat platelets conducted in Europe (euroSPRITE; see Table 6-3).[9] The study was carried out at four sites in the Netherlands, Swe-

Table 6-2. Platelet Counts and Bleeding Times in Thrombocytopenic Patients who Received Amotosalen-Treated Platelets*

	Pretransfusion (n = 10)	1-Hour Posttransfusion (n = 10)
Platelet count (× 10^6/µL)		
Control	14.5 ±6.3	52.3 ±18.3
PI platelets	13.2 ±5.3	41.9 ±20.8†
Corrected count increments (× 10^6/µL)		
Control	NA	13.6 ±4.3
PI platelets	NA	10.4 ±4.9‡
Bleeding time (minutes)		
Control	28.7 ±2.5	14.3 ±6.5
PI platelets	29.2 ±1.6	19.3 ±9.5

*Data from Slichter et al.[4,5]
†p = 0.007.
‡p <0.001.
PI = pathogen inactivation; NA = not applicable.

den, the United Kingdom, and France. Patients were those with hematologic malignancies, myelodysplasia, or solid tumors; about one-third were undergoing hematopoietic stem cell transplantation (Table 6-4). Patients with splenomegaly, a history of immune thrombocytopenia (ITP), disseminated intravascular coagulation (DIC), acute surgical conditions, platelet refractoriness, or pregnancy were excluded. For all platelet transfusions, the subjects were prospectively randomized to receive either buffy-coat-prepared platelets or buffy-coat platelets treated with amotosalen and UV for PI. The study involved all transfusions up to 8 weeks of platelet support if necessary, with an additional 4-week follow-up (Table 6-3). Platelets were ordered at each site by the attending physicians using a transfusion trigger of 20,000/µL. A total of 103 patients entered the

Table 6-3. Design of Clinical Trials of Pathogen-Inactivated Platelets

	euroSPRITE	SPRINT	MIRACLE
Type of platelets	Buffy coat	Amicus* apheresis	Apheresis and buffy coat
Study duration (weeks):	12	5	8
Transfusion period (weeks)	8	4	4
Surveillance period (weeks)	4	1	4
Primary endpoint	Count increment	Bleeding	Corrected count increment
Sample size	103	645	110
Number of sites	4	12	4
Age eligibility	≥12 years	≥6 years	≥16

*Fenwal, Lake Zurich, IL.

Table 6-4. Primary Diagnosis of Patients in Clinical Trials of Pathogen-Inactivated Platelets

	euroSPRITE (%)		SPRINT (%)		MIRACLE (%)	
	PI (n = 52)	Control (n = 51)	PI (n = 318)	Control (n = 327)	PI (n = 56)	Control (n-54)
Acute leukemia	50	47	28	26	50	54
Chronic leukemia	2	10	11	10	0	0
Lymphoma	0	0	24	29	35.7	39
Myelodysplasia	8	6	4	2	0	0
Plasma cell dyscrasia	0	0	20	18	7.1	3
Solid tumor	40	37	8	8	0	0
Other	0	0	6	4	7.2	4
Undergoing transplant	37	37	76	80	NA	NA

NA = not available.

trial and received at least one study transfusion. A total of 390 transfusions were given in the PI group and 256 transfusions in the control group (Table 6-5). Of these, 80% and 90%, respectively, were prepared according to the assigned protocol treatment arm. The PI and control platelets during the first eight transfusions resulted in different count increments (27.5 ±13.5 × 10^6/µL for PI vs 35.8 ±23.3 × 10^6/µL for control; $p = 0.03$; Table 6-5), but the PI platelet products contained fewer platelets (3.9 ±1.0 × 10^{11} vs 4.3 ±1.2 × 10^{11}; $p < 0.001$; Table 6-6). When the count increments were adjusted to take into account platelet dosage and the corrected count increment (CCI) was determined, the results were similar for both groups. The CCI for the PI group was 13.1 ±5.4 × 10^9, and for the control group, 14.9 ±6.2 × 10^9 ($p = 0.11$; Table 6-5).

When the results were examined by a longitudinal regression analysis for all transfusions, platelets subjected to PI had a 1-hour CCI that did not differ from the control platelets ($p = 0.53$; Fig 6-1). Thus, although there was a difference in the dose of platelets transfused between the PI and control groups, there was not a statistically significant difference between the CCIs of the two groups, and the linear regression model did not show a difference in the CCI for similar platelet doses between the two groups. However, because patients in the PI arm received a lower dose of platelets (3.9 vs 4.3 × 10^{11}; $p < 0.001$), they received a larger number of transfusions (7.5 vs 5.6; $p < 0.05$), and there was a trend toward a shorter time to the next transfusion (3.0 vs 3.4 days; Table 6-6).

There was no statistically significant difference in transfusion reactions between the two groups; however, the PI platelets were associated with a trend toward a lower rate of acute reactions compared to control platelets (1.6% vs 5%; $p = 0.61$). Overall, there was no difference in the incidence of adverse events. Serious adverse events were reported in 27% of patients who received PI platelets compared to 25% of patients who received control platelets (Table 6-7). The number of patients who died while on study (8%) was not different between the two groups, and none of the deaths were thought to be related to the study transfusions. In addition, hemorrhagic events were not different between the two groups (79% and 75%), nor were severe hemorrhagic events (6% in both groups; Table 6-7).

Thus, this study was very encouraging in that it established that, while posttransfusion platelet counts were lower in response to the

Table 6-5. Transfusion Results from Clinical Trials of Pathogen-Inactivated Platelets

	euroSPRITE		SPRINT		MIRACLE	
	PI	Control	PI	Control	PI	Control
Number of patients	52	51	318	327	56	54
Number of transfusions	390	256	2678	2041	368	310
Pretransfusion count ($\times 10^9$/L)	17	15	15	15	—	—
Posttransfusion count ($\times 10^9$/L)	44	50	36.5†	49.5	—	—
CI ($\times 10^9$/L)	27.5 ±3.5*	35.8 ±23.3	21†	34	—	—
CCI ($\times 10^9$)	13.1 ±5.4	14.9 ±6.2	11.1†	16.0	11.7	16.9‡

*First eight transfusions only; $p = 0.03$.
†$p < 0.001$.
‡$p < 0.001$.
CI = count increment; CCI = corrected count increment.

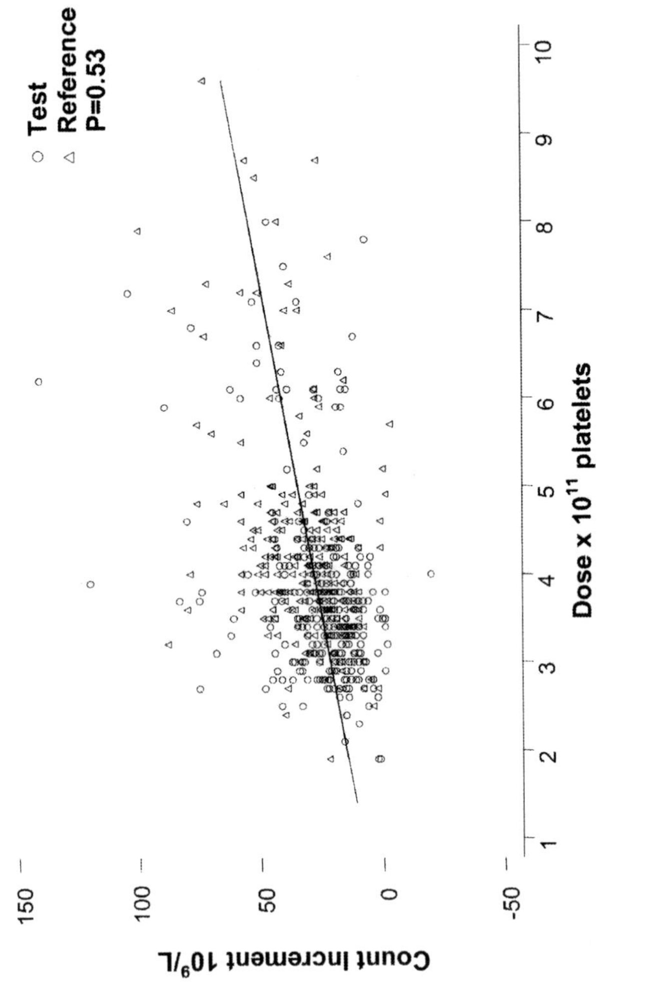

Figure 6-1. Effect of platelet dose on the 1-hour posttransfusion platelet count increment for test and control (reference) platelet transfusions. (Reprinted with permission from van Rhenen et al.[9])

Table 6-6. Platelet Use in Clinical Trials of Pathogen-Inactivated Platelets

	euroSPRITE		SPRINT		MIRACLE	
	PI (n = 52)	Control (n = 51)	PI (n = 318)	Control (n = 327)	PI (n = 56)	Control (n-54)
Number of transfusions	390	256	2678	2041	368	310
Mean number of transfusions	7.5*	5.6	8.4	6.2	4.5	3.0
Average platelet dose (× 10^{11})	3.9*	4.3	3.7*	4.0	2.9	3.0
Total platelet dose (× 10^{11})	22.3	21.2	29.4*	24.1	28.2	23.0
Number of transfusions per day of platelet support	0.49	0.44	0.74*	0.65	0.52	0.49
Average time between transfusions (days)	3.0	3.4	1.9*	2.4	2.2	2.3
Age of platelet concentrate (days)	3.5	3.4	3.4	3.6	2.8	2.6

*$p < 0.05$.

Table 6-7. Adverse Events in Clinical Trials of Pathogen-Inactivated Platelets*

	euroSPRITE		SPRINT		MIRACLE	
	PI	Control	PI	Control	PI	Control
Number of patients	52	51	318	327	56	54
Any AE (%)	100	100	99.7	98.2	100	98
Grade 3 or 4 AE (%)	—	—	78.9	78.6	67.8	55.6
Serious AE (%)	27	25	27	24.8	23.2	20.4
Treatment-related AE (%)	21	21	26	29	—	—
Death(%)	8	8	4	5	—	—
Any hemorrhagic AE						
Entire study (%)	85†	82†	90	85	80	56
Transfusion period (%)	79	75	83	75	—	—
Active surveillance (%)	24	35	31	33	—	—
Severe hemorrhagic AE (%)	6	6	23	20	11	5.6
Transfusion reaction (%)	1.6	5.0	3.0	4.4	—	—

*National Cancer Institute common toxicity criteria.
†$p < 0.05$.
AE = adverse event.

PI platelet products, there was not a significant difference in the CCI following transfusion when the dose of platelets was adjusted for consistency between the two groups, nor was there a documentable difference in the interval between transfusions. The overall occurrence and the nature of adverse events was similar between the two groups, and there was a suggestion that the rate of transfusion reactions might actually be reduced in those patients receiving PI platelets.

SPRINT

A larger study[10] was carried out at 12 sites in the United States with apheresis platelets subjected to PI using amotosalen and UV light, involving 645 patients (Table 6-3). Patients were assigned to receive either PI platelets or regular platelets, and platelets in both groups were collected with Amicus (Fenwal, Lake Zurich, IL) instrumentation. Patients remained on study for up to 4 weeks or until they became transfusion independent. Patients cytopenic as a result of chemotherapy or undergoing hematopoietic stem cell transplantation and expected to require at least two transfusions were entered in the study (Table 6-4). Patients were excluded if they had a positive lymphocytotoxic antibody test (>20% reactivity to a panel of cells), a history of platelet refractoriness, ITP, thrombotic thrombocytopenic purpura (TTP), acute promyelocyte leukemia, or recent surgery. Patients were randomized on a one-to-one basis to each arm, and all individuals involved in the clinical care and assessment of patients were blinded to the treatment assignment. (Blood bank and transfusion personnel responsible for randomization, collection, processing, and issue of platelets were not blinded.) This study was unique and groundbreaking in that it was the first clinical trial of platelet transfusions in which the primary endpoint was bleeding. The World Health Organization (WHO) bleeding scale (Table 6-8) was used, grading bleeding severity from 0 to 4. Hemostatic assessments were carried out daily. Each of eight potential bleeding sites (Table 6-9) was assigned a WHO bleeding grade, and the highest grade of any of the eight sites was the overall bleeding grade assigned for that day.

Platelet transfusions were given according to each institution's guidelines and the clinical decision of the attending physician but

Table 6-8. World Health Organization Bleeding Grades

Bleeding Grade	Type of Bleeding
0	None
1	Petechiae, ecchymosis, occult blood in body secretions, mild vaginal spotting
2	Evidence of gross hemorrhage not requiring red cell transfusion over routine transfusion needs (eg, epistaxis, hematuria, hematemesis)
3	Hemorrhage requiring transfusion of 1 or more units of red cells.
4	Life-threatening hemorrhage, defined as either massive bleeding causing hemodynamic compromise or bleeding into a vital organ (eg, intracranial, pericardial, or pulmonary hemorrhage)

Table 6-9. Body Systems Evaluated in the World Health Organization Bleeding Scale

Mucocutaneous
Gastrointestinal
Genitourinary
Broncho-pulmonary
Musculoskeletal and soft tissue
Body cavity
Central nervous system
Invasive sites

with a recommended threshold for prophylactic transfusion of 10,000/µL. ABO matching, use of irradiation, volume reduction, and HLA matching or crossmatching were all performed based on each institution's policies and the directives of the attending physicians.

A total of 671 patients were randomized; 645 of these received at least one platelet transfusion on study and composed the study population (Tables 6-4 and 6-5). The proportion of patients completing the transfusion period, the mean duration of platelet support (11.8 days PI vs 10.6 days control), and the proportion of patients achieving and maintaining platelet transfusion independence before day 28 (66% PI vs 70% control) were not different between the two treatment groups.[10] The study was designed as a noninferiority study; thus, the statistical tests were focused on determining whether the PI platelets produced an effect that was demonstrably not different from that of control platelets. The proportion of patients with Grade 2 or greater bleeding, which was the primary endpoint of the study, was not different in the PI group compared with the control group overall or for any of the eight potential bleeding sites (Table 6-10). For patients in the PI group, 58.5% experienced Grade 2 or greater bleeding compared with 57.5% of patients in the control group. The time to onset of the first episode of Grade 2 or greater bleeding after the beginning of the study did not differ significantly between the two groups (Fig 6-2). Also, there was no statistically significant difference between the two groups for Grade 3 or Grade 4 bleeding overall or for any of the eight potential bleeding sites (Table 6-10).

The mean 1-hour posttransfusion platelet increments were lower in the PI group (36.5×10^9/L) compared to the control group (49.5×10^9/L; $p < 0.001$; Table 6-5). When the platelet count increments were adjusted for platelet dose, the CCI was also different between the two groups (11.1×10^3 for PI vs 16.0×10^3 for control; $p < 0.001$; Table 6-5). However, patients in the PI group received a higher proportion of transfusions at doses less than 3×10^{11}. When patients receiving comparable doses of platelets were compared, there were no differences in the incidence or severity of bleeding or the number of platelet or red cell transfusions.[11]

The 645 patients in this study received a total of 4719 platelet transfusions (2678 PI vs 2041 control; Table 6-5). Thus, patients in the PI group received a larger mean number of platelet transfusions

Table 6-10. Proportion of Patients with Grade 2 or Higher Bleeding in the SPRINT Study

	PI: n (%) (n = 318)	Control: n (%) (n = 327)	p*
Any Grade 2 bleeding	186 (58.5)	188 (57.5)	<0.001†
Grade 2 bleeding by			
bleeding site	104 (32.7)	103 (31.5)	0.80
Genitourinary	82 (25.8)	65 (19.9)	0.08
Mucocutaneous	69 (21.7)	65 (19.9)	0.63
Invasive sites	60 (18.9)	63 (19.3)	0.92
Gastrointestinal	35 (11.0)	28 (8.6)	0.35
Respiratory	15 (4.7)	18 (5.5)	0.72
Musculoskeletal	0 (0.0)	1 (0.3)	1.00
Body cavity	0 (0.0)	0 (0.0)	—
Neurologic			
Any Grade 3 or 4 bleeding	13 (4.1)	20 (6.1)	<0.01‡

*Fisher exact test was used to calculate the p value for each of the eight potential bleeding sites.
†The P value for the overall proportion of patients with Grade 2 bleeding was <0.001, based on a noniferiority test with a noninferiority margin of 0.125 (one-sided 95% confidence interval of difference: –1, 0.07). By using this method, a p value of <0.05 indicates that pathogen inactivation was *not* inferior to control.
‡The p value for any Grade 3 or 4 bleeding was <0.01, based on a noniferiority test with a noniferiority margin of 0.07 (one-sided 95% confidence interval of difference: –1, 0.013). By using this method, a p value of <0.05 indicates that pathogen-inactivated platelets were not inferior to control.
(Data from McCullough et al.[10])

(8.4) compared to those in the control group (6.2; p <0.001). These differences might be at least partly explained by the lower dose of platelets received by patients in the PI group (3.7×10^{11} PI vs 4.0×10^{11} control; p <0.001). Other factors known to affect platelet re-

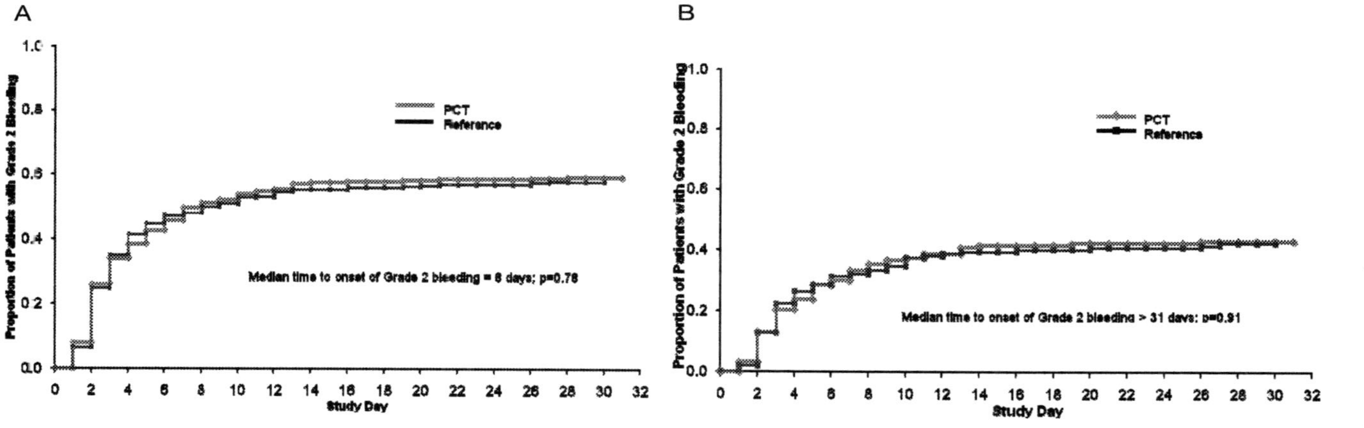

Figure 6-2. Median time to onset of Grade 2 bleeding. A: In intention-to-treat population (n = 645), 8 days; log-rank p = 0.78. B: In patients with no (Grade 0) bleeding at baseline (n = 541), more than 31 days; log-rank test p = 0.91. (Reprinted with permission from McCullough et al.[10])

covery, including average storage time, were not different between the two groups.

The differences in transfusion increment and CCI between the two groups was not surprising based on the Phase I studies of recovery and lifespan of radiolabeled pathogen inactivated platelets.[1] In that study, PI platelets prepared similarly to those used in the SPRINT and EuroSPRITE trials had a posttransfusion recovery of 42.5% compared to control, untreated platelets (50.3%; $p < 0.01$) and a lifespan of 4.8 days vs 6.0 days for controls ($p < 0.01$). Thus, it appears that the platelets treated with this PI technology are slightly damaged, leading to reduced posttransfusion recovery and survival, which could be expected to translate into a lower increment and CCI in clinical studies. However, it also appears that these PI platelets are as clinically effective as non-PI platelets in preventing or treating hemorrhage.[9-11] This concept has further support from the recent PLADO study examining the rate of bleeding in relation to the dose of platelets transfused.[12] In that study, the rate of bleeding remained generally constant in patients whose platelet counts ranged from 5000 to 80,000/µL. This is consistent with the observation that despite lower platelet count increments, the incidence of bleeding was similar in patients receiving either control or PI platelets.

Transfusion reactions were significantly less frequent following transfusion of PI platelets (3.0%) compared with control platelets (4.4%; $p = 0.02$), but there was no statistically significant difference in the proportion of patients who experienced the reaction (16.0% PI vs 19.3% control). Because these are very complex cases, most patients experienced some kind of adverse event (99.7% PI vs 98.2% control; Table 6-7). Grade 3 or 4 adverse events (78.9% PI, 78.6% control); serious adverse events (27.0% PI, 24.8% control); treatment-related adverse events (26.4% PI, 29.4% control); and deaths on study (3.5% PI, 5.2% control) were not different between the two groups (Table 6-7).

Adverse events were graded in severity using the National Cancer Institute common toxicity criteria[13] and coded using MedDRA, the medical dictionary for regulatory activities.[14] This resulted in a large number of categories of adverse events. Not surprisingly, when this large number of categories was compared, several of the categories showed significant differences between the PI and the control group. These adverse events were described in detail in a separate publication,[15] and most appeared to be small minor differences or not clinically significant. This further analysis of the SPRINT data showed that the overall safety of the amotosalen-treated platelets was comparable to untreated normal platelets, although the patients receiving PI platelets had petechiae statistically significantly more frequently, more fecal blood occult positivity, and more skin rashes.

Most of the categories of adverse events that were statistically significantly different showed higher rates of the events in the PI group, and a particular focus was placed by some regulators on acute respiratory distress syndrome, a complication that occurred in five patients in the PI group and none in the control group. Further detailed analysis by independent pulmonologists blinded to the treatment groups of 148 patients with any kind of pulmonary event revealed no significant differences between the groups for various pulmonary type adverse events (78% PI, 70% control).[15] Thus, while the differences in adverse events between the two groups did not suggest any major clinical problem, the predominance of statistically significantly higher adverse events in the PI group has led to concerns, particularly on the part of FDA, and this has resulted in hesitancy to approve the license application for this product in the United States despite the technique's acceptance in multiple European jurisdictions. Because platelets produced using this pathogen inactivation technique are widely used in Europe, considerable experience has accumulated. For example, in a report by Osselear et al,[16] 1400 patients received 7437 transfusions of platelets subjected to PI using the psoralen technology. In this noncontrolled observational study, 68 (0.9%) of the transfusions were associated with an adverse event, of which 55 (0.7%) were designated as possibly or probably related to the transfusion. Most were minor, and only 5 (0.07%) were classified as serious, but all were thought to be unrelated to the transfusion. The authors concluded that these PI platelets were well-tolerated in a wide range of patients.[16]

MIRACLE

The clinical trial MIRACLE evaluated platelets subjected to PI using the riboflavin plus UV light technology.[7] The trial[17] was carried out in four centers in France and was a prospectively randomized controlled trial comparing riboflavin-treated platelets with standard platelet products (Table 6-3). Patients in the trial were 16 years old or older and experiencing thrombocytopenia caused by chemotherapy, hematologic malignancy, or hematopoietic stem cell transplant (Table 6-4), and they were expected to receive at least two platelet transfusions as an inpatient. Patients were excluded if they were pregnant; had splenomegaly; had a history or diagnosis of autoimmune disease affecting hemostasis; had a history of refractoriness to platelet transfusion; revealed the presence of HLA antibodies or DIC; had a history of ITP, TTP, or HUS; or revealed the presence of other factors. The patient and attending physicians were not aware of the treatment arm to which the patient had been randomized and were blinded for the endpoint. (Blood center and transfusion service staff were aware of the treatment arm because they had to prepare the proper component.) The platelet units were prepared either by apheresis or the buffy-coat method, and thus patients in either treatment arm of the study might receive platelets produced via either or both approaches. Platelets were suspended in plasma and stored for up to 5 days but transfused after an average storage time of 2 to 3 days.

Patients received prophylactic platelet transfusions with a platelet count of 10,000/μL or below unless there were clinical complicating factors, such as fever, that would support the use of a 20,000/μL platelet-count threshold. Patients remained on study for 4 weeks, with an additional 4 week follow-up.

The primary endpoint in this study was the 1-hour CCI of the first eight transfusions. This was designed as a noninferiority study, so the objective was to show that the outcomes from using PI platelets were not different from using control platelets.

The centers enrolled 118 patients, although four patients in each treatment group did not receive platelet transfusions, and thus 110 patients formed the intent-to-treat group in this trial. Ten patients (6 PI, 4 control) withdrew from the study before completion. The reasons for this were as follows: withdrew consent, 2 (PI); death, 4 (3 PI, 1 control); final selection criteria not fulfilled, 3 (control); and other, 1 (PI). The proportion of patients who completed the treatment period was similar for the two groups (91% PI, 98% control), and the proportion of patients completing the second 28-day follow-up for safety evaluation also was similar between the two groups (73%, PI, 81% control).

The patients in the two groups were similar in terms of age, gender, size, ABO blood group distribution, diagnosis, and baseline complete blood counts. About one-half of the patients in the study had acute myelogenous leukemia, and an additional one-third, non-Hodgkin lymphoma, with patients similarly distributed between the two groups (Table 6-4).

A total of 678 platelet transfusions were given to patients during this study—368 to the PI group and 310 to the control group (Tables 6-5 and 6-11). There was a substantial incidence of off-protocol transfusions (17.7% PI, 23.2% control). The reasons for the off-protocol transfusions were not specified.

The primary endpoint of 1-hour CCI was based on a total of 467 transfusions (258 PI, 209 control). The mean CCI for the PI group was 11,725 and the control group, 16,939 (Table 6-11). Statistical analysis of these data does not allow the claim of noninferiority; in other words, the data do not support the conclusion that the CCI from the PI group was the same as that from the controls. However, this statistical method does not establish that the PI group was different or inferior, because that was not the structure of the study and neither were such statistical methods used. Similar results occur

Table 6-11. Key Results of the MIRACLE Trial of Platelets Pathogen Inactivated Using Riboflavin

	Control	PI
Patients (n)	54	56
Transfusions—total	310	368
Transfusions—evaluable	209	258
Platelet count pretransfusion ($\times 10^6/\mu L$) CCI	16,939	11,725*
Transfusion interval (days)	2.3	2.2
Number transfusions/patient	3.0	4.5
Total platelet dose ($\times 10^{11}$)	23.0	28.2
Alloimmunized (%)	7.4	2.6
Bleeding > WHO Grade 2 (%)	56	80
Grade 2 (patients)	5	11
Grade 3 (patients)	2	4
Grade 4 (patients)	1	2
Death	1	3

*$p < 0.001$.
CCI = corrected count increment; WHO = World Health Organization.

when the CCI is calculated based only on the platelet counts that were obtained within the predesignated time period surrounding the transfusion.[17] As the authors to this study point out,[17] "although the mean CCI values for both 1 and 24 hours were lower with pathogen inactivated product, the values for both determinations were above the 7500 and 4500 thresholds used to define successful transfusions."

There were no statistically significant differences between the two groups for the following secondary objectives: mean number of days between platelet transfusions (2.2 PI, 2.3 control); percentage of transfusions that were apheresis vs buffy coat; mean number of platelet transfusions per patient (4.5 PI, 3.0 control); mean number of transfusions per day on study (0.52 PI, 0.49 control); average total dose of platelets transfused (28.2×10^{11} PI vs 23.0×10^{11} control; $p = 0.13$); and average number of platelets transfused per meter squared of body surface area (2.91 PI, 3.01 control) when all transfusions—including those off protocol—were considered.

Only two patients in the PI group became alloimmunized (2.6%), compared with four patients in the control group (7.4%). Bleeding assessments were performed both before and after transfusion for all transfusions given on protocol. Bleeding equal to or greater than WHO Grade 2 occurred in 45 patients in the PI arm (80%) and 30 patients in the control group (56%; $p > 0.05$; see Table 6-11). For Grades 3 and 4, there were no statistically significant differences between the PI and control patients (Table 6-11). Patients in this study were extremely ill, and almost all had at least one adverse event (98.1% PI, 100% control).

Recent Clinical Studies

Intersol/Intercept Study

In this three-arm study, 68 patients received platelets stored in plasma (PL), 64 received platelets stored in Intersol (Fenwal Inc., Lake Zurich, IL) platelet additive solution (PAS), and 67 received platelets stored in Intersol and subjected to PI with the psoralen technology (PAS/PI).[18] An interim analysis report included only 135 of 199 evaluable patients and from only the PL and PAS/PI arms of the study. The number of patients in each group was not reported. There was a statistically significant difference in the 1-hour CCI: 11.4 ±5.4 for PAS/PI vs 17.5 ±7.1 × $10^6/\mu L$ for PL ($p < 0.0001$). Bleeding episodes were more common in the PAS/PI patients compared to the PL patients ($p = 0.045$). Unfortunately neither the type of bleeding nor the incidence were reported. Thus, while the data are provocative, it will be important to see the extensive data when it is available in a full manuscript.

Seven-Day Intercept Study

Cerus has recently announced completion of a study comparing increments in 6- and 7-day stored additive platelets with and without Intercept treatment, claiming noninferiority in increments.[19]

UVC-Treated Platelets

Pathogen inactivation of platelets using UVC light with no other additions is also under development.[20-22] Initial Phase I clinical trials are being initiated, but data are not available at the time of this writing.

Dutch-Belgian HOVON Group

This three arm study compared buffy coat platelets stored in plasma or stored in platelet additive solution (PASIII) or subjected to pathogen reduction (PR-PASIII) using the Intercept method and stored in platelet additive solution (23). Platelets were stored for seven days. A total of 278 patients were randomized into the three study groups: plasma = 99, PASIII = 94, and PR-PASIII = 85. The primary endpoint was the one-hour corrected count increment with the study designed as noninferiority comparing PASIII and PR-PASIII with plasma. This seems odd because it was well established that Intercept platelets give lower CCIs than untreated platelets. Also, while bleeding was one of several secondary endpoints, the publically available protocol does not include any description of bleeding assessments and also it appears that this study was not blinded. For the primary endpoint, the CCIs were significantly for the PR-PASIII group than the other two groups (p value not given). While this merely confirmed previous information, the disturbing finding was an increase in the number of patients who experience bleeding in the PR-PASIII arm (32%) compared to the plasma (19% and PASIII (15%) arms ($p = 0.034$). The authors also report higher grade bleeding in the PR-PASIII group (0.044). There was no difference in bleeding site and no fatal bleeding occurred during the study. There were no differences in red cell transfusions, platelet dose, storage time, gamma irradiation, or transfusion reactions. These results must be viewed in light of the study design.

References

1. Snyder E, Raife T, Lin L, et al. Recovery and life span of ^{111}indium-radiolabeled platelets treated with pathogen inactivation with amotosalen HCl (S-59) and ultraviolet A light. Transfusion 2004;44:1732-40.
2. Lin L, Cook DN, Wiesehahn JP, et al. Photochemical inactivation of viruses and bacateria in platelet concentrates by use of a novel psoralin and long-wavelength ultraviolet light. Transfusion 1997;37:423-35.
3. Pineda A, McCullough J, Benjamin RJ, et al. Pathogen inactivation of platelets using a photochemical treatment with amotosalen HC1 and ultraviolet light: Process used in the SPRINT trial. Transfusion 2006;46:562-71.
4. Slichter SJ, Corash L, Grabowski M, et al. Viability and hemostatic function of photochemically-treated platelets in thrombocytopenic patients (abstract). Blood 1999;94:376a.
5. Slichter SJ, Raife TJ, Davis K, et al. Platelets photochemically treated with amotosalen HCl and ultraviolet A light correct prolonged bleeding times in patients with thrombocytopenia. Transfusion 2006;46:731-40.
6. Goodrich RP, Li J, Edrich R, Seghatchian J. The Mirasol PRT system for pathogen reduction of platelets and plasma: An overview of current status and future trends. Transfus Apher Sci 2006;35:5-17.
7. Goodrich RP. The use of riboflavin for the inactivation of pathogens in blood products. Vox Sang 2000;78:211-15.
8. AuBuchon JP, Herschel L, Roger J, et al. Efficacy of apheresis platelets treated with riboflavin and ultraviolet light for pathogen reduction. Transfusion 2005; 45:1335-41.
9. van Rhenen D, Gulliksson H, Cazenave JP, et al. Transfusion of pooled buffy coat platelet components prepared with photochemical pathogen inactivation treatment: The euroSPRITE trial. Blood 2003;101:2426-33.
10. McCullough J, Vesole DH, Benjamin RJ, et al. Therapeutic efficacy and safety of platelets treated with a photochemical process for pathogen inactivation: The SPRINT trial. Blood 2004;104:1534-41.

11. Murphy S, Snyder E, Cable R, et al for the SPRINT study group. Platelet dose consistency and its effect on the number of platelet transfusions for support of thrombocytopenia: An analysis of the SPRINT trial of platelet photochemically-treated with amotosalen HCL and ultraviolet A light. Transfusion 2006; 46:24-33.
12. Slichter SJ, Kaufman RM, Assmann SF, et al. Dose of prophylactic platelet transfusions and prevention of hemorrhage. N Engl J Med 2010;362:600-13.
13. Trotti A, Byhardt R, Stetz J, et al. Common toxicity criteria version 2.0. An improved reference for grading the acute effects of cancer treatment: Impact of radiotherapy. Int J Radiat Oncol Biol Phys 2000;47:13-47.
14. Medical dictionary for regulatory activities. MedDRA introductory guide. Version 3.3 (December 2002). Reston, VA: Maintenance and Support Services Organization, 2002.
15. Snyder E, McCullough J, Slichter SJ, et al. Clinical safety of platelets photochemically treated with amotosalen HC1 and ultraviolet A light for pathogen inactivation: The SPRINT trial. Transfusion 2005;45:1864-75.
16. Osselaer JC, Cazenave JP, Lambermount M, et al. An active haemovigilance programme characterizing the safety profile of 7437 platelet transfusions prepared with amotosalen photochemical treatment. Vox Sang 2008;94:315-23.
17. MIRACLE study group. A randomized controlled trial evaluating the performance and safety of platelets treated with MIRASOL pathogen reduction technology. Transfusion (in press).
18. Kerkhoffs JH, Novotny VM, Boekhorst PAT, et al. Clinical effectiveness and safety of pooled, random donor platelet concentrates, leucoreduced and stored up to seven days in either plasma or additive solution with and without pathogen reduction in hemato-oncological patients (abstract). Transfusion 2009;49:2A.
19. Cerus Corporation reports positive outcome in European study of 7-Day Intercept Platelets (press release). (January 14, 2010) Concord, CA: Cerus, 2010.
20. Terpstra FG, van 't Wout AB, Schuitemaker H, et al. Potential and limitation of UVC irradiation for the inactivation of pathogens in platelet concentrates. Transfusion 2008;48:304-13.
21. Mohr H, Gravemann U, Bayer A, Müller TH. Sterilization of platelet concentrates at production scale by irradiation with short-wave ultraviolet light. Transfusion 2009;49:1956-63.
22. Mohr H, Steil L, Gravemann U, et al. A novel approach to pathogen reduction in platelet concentrates using short-wave ultraviolet light. Transfusion 2009;49:2612-24.
23. Kerkoffs JLH, van Putten WLJ, Novotny VMJ, et al. Clinical effectiveness of leucoreduced, pooled donor platelet concentrates, stored in plasma or additive solution with and without pathogen reduction. Br J Haematol 2010;150: 209-17.

In: AuBuchon JP, Prowse CV, eds.
Pathogen Inactivation: The Penultimate Paradigm Shift
Bethesda, MD: AABB Press, 2010

7

Norway: Solvent/Detergent Plasma

BJARTE G. SOLHEIM, MD, PHD, MHA, AND
ØYSTEIN FLESLAND MD, PHD

NORWAY IS A SPARSELY POPULATED COUNTRY WITH 4.8 million inhabitants. Blood donation is voluntary and nonremunerated, and all blood banks are hospital associated. Self-sufficiency had been the national goal from 1980 until 2009, when it was decided that Norwegian plasma should be sold on the open market. The more-than-50 Norwegian blood banks produce in total 50 to 60 tons of plasma per year, of which approximately 90% has been recovered plasma. Over 95% of the plasma has been frozen within 4 to 8 hours after collection.

Bjarte G. Solheim, MD, PhD, MHA, Professor Emeritus, Institute of Immunology, Oslo University Hospital—Rikshospitalet and University of Oslo, and Øystein Flesland MD, PhD, Director, National Patient Safety Unit, Norwegian Knowledge Centre for the Health Services, Oslo, Norway

The authors have disclosed no conflicts of interest.

In the first part of the 1980s, the policy of self-sufficiency and use of cryoprecipitate and Factor IX prepared from small plasma pools resulted in a prevalence of antibodies to the human immunodeficiency virus (HIV) of only 6% in the Norwegian hemophilia population.[1] Because of the HIV epidemic, the Norwegian health authorities decided in 1985 that plasma, cryoprecipitate, and Factor IX should be replaced by virus-inactivated products prepared from Norwegian plasma. Virus-inactivated coagulation factors were introduced by 1988, while plasma consumption was reduced to a minimum until a suitable method for virus inactivation of fresh frozen plasma (FFP) became available.

Because plasma production in Norway is insufficient for the establishment of a fractionation plant, the Norwegian Plasma Fractionation Project was initiated by the blood banks. Based on tenders on the European market, this project began in 1988 to coordinate delivery of plasma and the return of fractionated and/or virus-inactivated blood components for use in hospitals and distribution by the Institute for Haemophilia for home treatment.[2] From 1988 through 2005, Octapharma AG (Lachen, Switzerland) won the bid and performed the fractionation and/or virus inactivation of Norwegian plasma until June 2009. Production was carried out at Octapharma's plants in Vienna, Austria, and for the last couple of years, in part in Stockholm, Sweden. [An exception was the test fractionation in 1988 and part of 1989, when fractionation was performed at Centre Regional de Transfusion Sanguine (CRTS) in Lille, France.] The fractionation project was ended in 2009 by the Norwegian health trusts owning the hospitals. The process leading to this decision has not been transparent but appears to be based on considerations such as the health trusts' decision that all plasma products were equally safe. The question of whether plasma should come from paid or nonremunerated donors was not considered or was considered irrelevant in spite of the fact that Norway has endorsed the Council of Europe's principle of voluntary, nonremunerated blood donation. In addition, the health trusts desired a simpler system, even if the result would be higher total costs for health care. The result is that now plasma is sold to the highest bidder. Plasma products based on foreign plasma are imported and distributed by the health trusts' pharmacies. Solvent/detergent (SD) plasma from foreign plasma is imported by the health trusts and distributed by the blood banks.

Introduction and Logistics

In 1991-1992 it became clear that plasma could be virally inactivated by methylene blue and visible light illumination or SD treatment.[3-5] Because of extensive documentation of the SD method, favorable experience with SD treatment of plasma products, and the Norwegian contract fractionation agreement with Octapharma, a clinical study with SD-treated plasma (Octaplas) was performed at Rikshospitalet, University Hospital, Oslo in 1992.[6] The study was performed with 200-mL units of lyophilized Octaplas and demonstrated that the product was effective, but the clinicians expressed preference for frozen instead of lyophilized plasma. After conclusion of the clinical study and in accordance with the decision in 1985 to substitute FFP with a virally inactivated product, the health authorities decided that Octaplas should be substituted for FFP. Bags of 200 mL frozen SD plasma were to be produced from Norwegian plasma. In order to simplify logistics, production was limited to blood group A and group AB plasma (group A plasma to be transfused to group A and O patients; AB plasma to AB and B patients and emergency cases with unknown ABO type). The plan to introduce SD plasma early in 1993 was delayed by the loss of the first three batches in a ferry accident, but by June 1993 the switch to SD plasma was completed in Norway.

From 1993 to 2009, 588,652 units of Octaplas were produced from Norwegian plasma for blood banks in Norway. Now, after termination of the plasma fractionation project, consumption in Norway is based on Octaplas produced from Western European plasma. The prion-reduced OctaplasLG, which has plasmin inhibitor within the normal range, replaces Octaplas in 2010. For safety and logistic reasons, a switch to prion-reduced universal plasma [Uniplas (Octapharma)] will probably follow after the product has been licensed. A successful clinical study in open-heart surgery has been performed in Norway with Uniplas.[7]

Except for about 1000 units of methylene-blue/light-treated plasma produced for clinical studies in 2002 and a few hundred units of quarantine plasma, only SD plasma has been used in Norway since its introduction in 1993. The costs for methylene blue plasma and quarantine plasma proved to be on the same magnitude as those for SD plasma.

Changes in the Use of Plasma Colloids

Before 1985, there was considerable use of cryo-depleted plasma in Norway, but in the following years it reduced rapidly. At the same time, the previously modest use of FFP increased (Fig 7-1). From 1989 until 1993, the annual consumption maintained stability around 4400 units FFP per million inhabitants. After the introduction of SD plasma, the consumption increased gradually, and by 2009 it had increased 130% to 10,129 units SD plasma per million inhabitants. However, the introduction of SD plasma reduced the unit volume from 270 mL to 200 mL; thus the consumed FFP volume increased only 71%, representing a plasma consumption of 2026 L per million inhabitants. This is below the mean consumption of 2368 L per million inhabitants in Western Europe but well above countries such as France, the Netherlands, Ireland, and the United Kingdom that use plasma in the range of 1172 to 1723 L per million inhabitants [C. L. van der Poel, Sanquin (organization in the Netherlands), personal communication]. After 1985, the albumin consumption increased significantly (Fig 7-1) and peaked in 1989 with 332.9 kg albumin/million inhabitants. In the following years the consumption of albumin decreased gradually until it had a marked drop after publication of the Cochrane Group report in 1998.[8] Since 2001, the consumption has been reduced only from 120 to 107 kg/million inhabitants.

System Changes as a Result of the Introduction of SD Plasma

Because of its adequate content of clotting factors and very low residual concentration of solvent and detergent, SD plasma was introduced in 1993 for all patients in need of plasma, including neonates and liver transplant patients, and for exchange transfusions.

In a clinical study performed at Rikshospitalet in 1994-95 to identify possible risk factors associated with transfusion of large volumes of SD plasma, 1170 patients undergoing 1201 consecutive open-heart operations were studied (898 adults and 272 children). The study demonstrated that SD plasma was effective and caused very few side effects even after transfusion of up to 18 L in adults

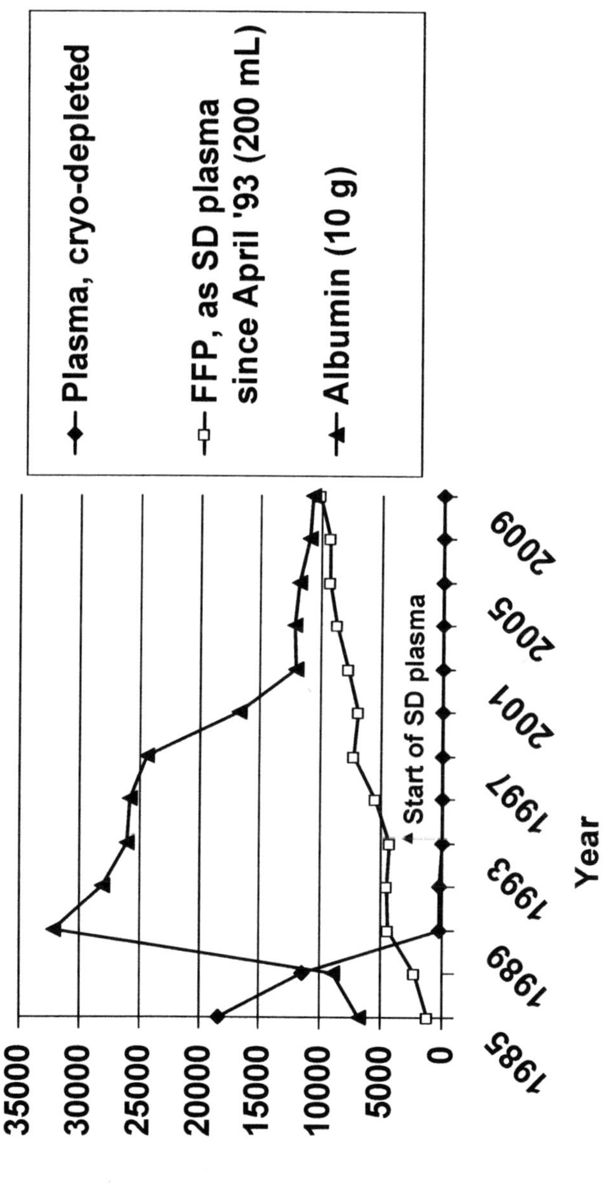

Figure 7-1. Plasma and albumin usage in Norway from 1985 to 2009. FFP = fresh frozen plasma; SD = solvent/detergent.

and 2 to 3 L in children. SD plasma was also found to be safe with regard to lipid-enveloped viruses and showed that immune antibodies are of importance in avoiding clinical disease with the nonenveloped viruses hepatitis A and parvovirus B19.[9]

So far over 620 liver transplants have been performed at Rikshospitalet, University Hospital, Oslo using SD plasma as the only plasma component, with good effect. No cases of thromboembolism have been ascribed to its use. Because of the low content of plasmin inhibitor in Octaplas, aprotinin was often used in severe liver failure and complicated repeat cardiac surgery.[10] Now aprotinin has been successfully substituted with the anti-fibrinolytic drug tranexamic acid in cardiac surgery and liver transplantation, except in some very few liver transplant patients in need of a broad-spectrum serine protease inhibitor.

SD plasma volumes equalling 30% of body weight were well tolerated by both neonates and adults on extracorporeal membrane oxygenator treatment during 3- to 6-week treatment periods. SD plasma has also successfully been used in more than 500 plasma exchanges, where it proved to reduce allergic reactions significantly.

The initial use of SD plasma for emergency reversal of warfarin treatment has partly been replaced by prothrombin complex concentrate [Octaplex (Octapharma)] since 2002.

The attributes of the SD plasma product—ie, it is well tolerated, has a predictable effect as a result of standardized protein content and activity, is produced in a standardized 200-mL volume,[11] and is a clear solution—have made it popular, particularly among surgeons and anesthesiologists. This, in combination with the increasing complexity of patient treatment, is the main explanation for the escalation in plasma consumption.

Costs

The cost of SD plasma is the cost or value of the plasma and SD treatment, including transportation costs. From 1993 until 2007, the price for a unit of Octaplas (200 mL SD plasma) issued from the blood banks was 455 Norwegian Krones (NOK 455 = ~US$76, €54—based on an exchange rate of NOK 6 = ~US$1 and NOK 8.5 = ~€1), while the plasma delivered by the blood banks (for fractionation/SD-treatment) was valued at slightly over NOK 1000

(US$167, ∈118) per liter of delivered plasma.[2] Since 2008, the price has been NOK 497 (US$83, ∈58) for a unit of Octaplas, which increased the value of plasma delivered (for fractionation/SD-treatment) to approximately NOK 1200 (US$200, ∈142) per liter of plasma. The total extra costs for a 200-mL SD plasma unit have thus been approximately NOK 255 (US$43, ∈30).

Hemovigilance

Since its introduction in Norway in 1993, Octaplas has been classified as a pharmaceutical product. Its use thus confers an obligation to report serious adverse events to the Norwegian Medicines Agency. So far, only two such events have been reported. In 1993, 800 mL of SD plasma were transfused rapidly to an elderly patient for volume expansion, resulting in arrhythmia and cardiac arrest. The patient was resuscitated and recovered completely. In 2004, a serious anaphylactic reaction occurred after transfusion of 400 mL SD plasma. The patient subsequently recovered completely.

Since 2004, Norway has had a national hemovigilance system with very high participation. All types of transfusion reactions are reported, not only the serious ones.[12] The hemovigilance data (Table 7-1) show that transfusion reactions caused by Octaplas are reported at a rate of 27 per 100,000 transfused units, compared to 144 per 100,000 transfused red cell units and 369 per 100,000 transfused platelet units. In contrast, in the Danish hemovigilance system, FFP is the product that gives the highest rate of transfusion reactions.[13] If these systems are comparable, the use of Octaplas may have saved approximately 340 transfusion reactions per 100,000 transfusions. There has been no viral transmission by Octaplas in Norway,[14] nor has there been any report of transfusion-related acute lung injury (TRALI) caused by Octaplas, although on average one case of TRALI caused by red cell or platelet transfusions is reported annually. This is interesting compared to Swedish hemovigilance data showing 38 reports of TRALI between 2004 and 2007, of which plasma was involved in 31.[15] Because Sweden has almost twice the population of Norway, this may suggest that 15 patients in Norway were saved from TRALI in a 4-year period, or 60 patients in 16 years, by the use of Octaplas.

Table 7-1. Blood Products Involved in Transfusion Reactions in Norway

	2004	2005	2006	2007	2008	Total 2004-08	Adverse Events/100,000 units, 2004-08
Red cells	259	195	255	342	341	1392	143.9
Platelets	44	41	52	93	96	326	369.0
Octaplas*	6	13	10	15	14	58	27.4
Other	4	8	4	9	6	31	
Not specified	2	3	16	1	2	24	
Total	315	260	337	460	459	1831	

*Octapharma AG, Lachen, Switzerland.

The reported transfusion reactions have mostly been mild, nonhemolytic febrile reactions and mild allergic reactions. Since 2004 there have been only five reports of severe allergic reactions in >210,000 transfusions. (One of them was also significant enough to be reported to the Norwegian Medicines Agency.) There has been one report of incompatible Octaplas transfused as a result of a mix-up of patient identity where blood group A plasma was transfused to a group B patient without immediate problems, but subsequently the patient experienced slight hemoglobinemia.

The fact that transfusion of SD plasma results in very few transfusion reactions is important because even a mild transfusion reaction, in addition to being uncomfortable for the patient, often delays necessary transfusions, may cause products to be discarded, and results in extra work in the blood bank and on the ward.

In order to simplify logistics, Norway has chosen to transfuse group A Octaplas to group A and O patients, and AB Octaplas to AB, B, and emergency patients. Because Shanwell and collaborators have reported increased posttransfusion mortality among group O patients receiving AB plasma but not in other recipients of ABO-compatible but nonidentical plasma,[16] the authors analyzed over 40,000 Octaplas transfusions at Rikshospitalet, University Hospital, Oslo. No increased mortality was observed after transfusion of A Octaplas to O patients or AB Octaplas to B patients. Neither was there observed increased mortality after transfusion of AB Octaplas in emergency situations to O, A, or B patients. However, there were few group O patients receiving AB plasma. Taking Shanwell's data into account, a national analysis of AB Octaplas transfusions should be carried out. This is particularly important because many small hospitals have chosen to use only AB Octaplas in order to increase safety and simplify logistics.

Conclusion

Norway has 16 years experience with the SD plasma Octaplas as the only frozen plasma for transfusion. Octaplas has been used in all kinds of patients, including neonates, and in all kinds of procedures, including more than 620 liver transplants. It has proved to be safe, effective, and easy to use. Compared to FFP, the cost has increased by about 100%, but the savings have also been substantial when avoided transfusion reactions, including TRALI, are included in the calculation.

References

1. Evensen SA, Ulstrup J, Skaug K, et al. HIV infection in Norwegian haemophiliacs: The prevalence of antibodies against HIV in heamophiliacs treated with lyophilized cryoprecipitate from volunteer donors. Eur J Haematol 1987; 39:44-8.
2. Flesland O, Seghatchian J, Solheim BG. The Norwegian plasma fractionation project—a 12 year clinical and economic success story. Transfus Apher Sci 2003;28:93-100.
3. Lambrecht B, Mohr H, Knüver-Hopf J, Schmitt H. Photoinactivation of viruses in human plasma by phenothiazine dyes in combination with visible light. Vox Sang 1991;60:207-13.
4. Horowitz B, Bonomo R, Prince AM, et al. Solvent/detergent-treated plasma. A virus-inactivated substitute for fresh frozen plasma. Blood 1992;79:826-33.
5. Hellstern P, Sachse H, Schwinn H, Oberefrank K. Manufacture and in-vitro characterization of a solvent/detergent-treated plasma. Vox Sang 1992;63: 178-85.
6. Solheim BG, Svennevig JL, Mohr B, et al. The use of Octaplas in patients undergoing open heart surgery. In: Müller-Berghaus G, Madlener K, Blombäck M, Ten Cate JW, eds. DIC pathogenesis and disseminated intravascular fibrin formation. Amsterdam: Experta Medica, Elsevier Science Publishers, 1993: 253-62.
7. Tølløfsrud S, Noddeland H, Svennevig JL, et al. Universal fresh frozen plasma (Uniplas): A safe product in open-heart surgery. Intensive Care Med 2003;29:1736-43.
8. Cochrane Injuries Group Albumin Reviewers. Human albumin administration in critically ill patients: Systematic review of randomised controlled trials. BMJ 1998;317:235-40.
9. Solheim BG, Rollag H, Svennevig JL, et al. Viral safety of solvent/detergent-treated plasma. Transfusion 2000;40:84-90.
10. Solheim BG, Bergan A, Brosstad F, et al. Fibrinolysis during liver transplant and use of solvent/detergent virus-inactivated plasma (ESDEP/Ocatplas) (letter). Anesth Analg 2003;96:1230-1.
11. Beeck H, Hellstern P. In vitro characterization of solvent/detergent treated human plasma and of quarantine fresh frozen plasma. Vox Sang 1998; 74(Suppl 1):219-23.
12. Hemovigilans. (For Norwegian hemovigilance reports.) Oslo, Norway: Nasjonalt kunnskapssenter for helsetjenesten, 2010. [Available at http://www.hemovigilans.no.]

13. DART Haemovigilancerapport for 2007. (For Danish hemovigilance report.) [Available at http://www.haemovigilance.dk/pdf/DART_2007.pdf (accessed May 3, 2010).]
14. Flesland O. A comparison of complication rates based on published haemovigilance data. Intensive Care Med 2007;33(Suppl 1):S17-21.
15. Blodövervakning under 2004-2007. (For Swedish hemovigilance report.) [Available at http://www3.svls.se/sektioner/tr/Arkiv/Blodverksamhet%20i%20Sverige/Blodovervakning2004-2007.pdf (accessed May 3, 2010).]
16. Shanwell A, Andersson TML, Rostgaard K, et al. Post-transfusion mortality among recipients of ABO-compatible but non-identical plasma. Vox Sang 2009;96:316-24.

In: AuBuchon JP, Prowse CV, eds.
Pathogen Inactivation: The Penultimate Paradigm Shift
Bethesda, MD: AABB Press, 2010

8

France: Solvent/Detergent Plasma

GEORGES ANDREU, MD, PHD

THE SOLVENT/DETERGENT (SD) METHOD TO INACTIVATE enveloped viruses in therapeutic plasma (SD plasma) was developed in the 1980s, and its effectiveness in inactivating major enveloped viruses was immediately recognized.[1-6] SD treatment of plasma had been initially conceived as a process similar to most plasma-derived drugs—ie, prepared from recovered plasma in large pools of a thousand donations or more. In 1991, the French health authorities were reluctant to license SD plasma, fearing that such a product could cause widespread dissemination of any infectious agent

Georges Andreu, MD, PhD, Councelor of the General Director, Institut National de la Transfusion Sanguine, Paris, France

The author has disclosed no conflicts of interest.

insensitive to SD treatment and either completely unknown or known but with no available diagnostic test for blood donors. However, as the ability of this process to inactivate enveloped viruses was acknowledged, it was considered useful to introduce such a product in France. The final decision was to authorize the manufacturing of SD plasma in France in pools of a maximum of a hundred donations of the same ABO blood group.

This constraint led to the choice of plasma collected by apheresis as the source for SD plasma, with a maximal collection of 600 mL of plasma (plus anticoagulant; ie, about 650 mL of initial material) per donation in order to prepare batches of about 60 L, the final product being issued in bags of 200 mL. In addition, in order to maximize Factor VIII preservation, these plasma units are frozen within 6 hours of collection. In 1992, a single blood transfusion center located in Bordeaux was authorized to produce SD plasma in France. This situation remains unchanged since that time.

The manufacturing process for SD plasma in France is summarized in Table 8-1.

Table 8-1. Manufacturing Process for SD Plasma

Preinactivation Step
- Selection of a maximum of 100 plasma units collected by apheresis with the same ABO blood group, with the following exclusion criteria:
  - Positive nucleic acid testing for parvovirus B19
  - Hemolysis or hyperlipemia after thawing
- Pooling, clarifying filtration, and introduction into a vat

Inactivation Step
- Introduction of 1% tri-n-butyl phosphate (TNBP) and Triton X-100
- Incubation for 4 hours at 30 C

Elimination of TNBP and Triton X-100
- Addition of castor oil
- Two consecutive filtrations
- Chromatography

Final Steps
- Sterilizing filtration (0.22 µm)
- Sterile dispensing in bags of 200 mL
- Freezing

Quality Controls

The quality control (QC) procedures performed on every blood donation in France include ABO, Rh1, -2, -3, -4, and -5, and Kell1 phenotyping; red cell alloantibody screening; high-titer A and B antibody determination; full blood count (hemoglobin, red cells, platelets, and leukocytes); syphilis screening; tests for hepatitis B surface antigen, hepatitis B core antibody, antibody to human immunodeficiency virus (HIV) types 1 and 2, antibody to human T-cell lymphotropic virus types 1 and 2, and antibody to hepatitis C virus (HCV); nucleic acid testing (NAT) for HIV and HCV; and testing for antibody to plasmodia and/or *Trypanosoma cruzi* (when required by donor characteristics). Additional tests are performed specifically on plasma donors for SD plasma production.

Quality Control Procedures Performed Before Pooling

Since 2005, the European Pharmacopoeia monograph regarding plasma pools for viral inactivation requires systematic parvovirus B19 NAT testing. This is particularly pertinent in the case of SD plasma, as this inactivation process is not efficient against nonenveloped viruses. Parvovirus B19 NAT screening is performed using an in-house method in pools of 96 plasma units. In any plasma pool identified as positive, the units are subsequently individually tested with the Parvo B19 LC PCR Artus test (Artus Biotech USA, San Francisco, CA). Every unit found with a positivity equal to or above the 10.0-IU/µL control prepared from the European Pharmacopoeia standard (titled "B19 Virus DNA BRP Batch 1") is discarded. This testing results in the elimination of 0.08% of donations.[7]

Quality Control Procedures Performed After Elimination of TNBP and Triton X-100

Factor VIII Concentration

In France, every therapeutic plasma unit should contain a minimum of 0.7 IU of Factor VIII per mL. This specification may be difficult to obtain for SD plasma, despite a careful management of the initial freezing after collection, especially in group O plasma. In the French experience, after elimination of TNBP and Triton X-100, about 50% of group O batches contain less than 0.7 IU of Factor VIII (mean = 0.71 IU/mL), while ABO groups A, B, and AB have much better results (group A: 4% of batches <0.7 IU/mL, mean = 0.83; group B: 6% <0.7 IU/mL, mean = 0.86; and group AB: 6% <0.7 IU/mL, mean = 0.86).[7] Therefore at this step, after Factor VIII concentration analysis, an additional concentration step by dialysis may be added if needed. This additional step enables the production of SD plasma batches with Factor VIII concentrations complying with the French regulation.[8]

HLA and Granulocyte Antibody Testing

Each pool is tested before release for HLA[9] and granulocyte (leukoagglutination) antibodies.[10] Since 1992, only one positive pool has been found, and it was discarded.

Parvovirus B19 Postelimination Testing

Each pool of SD plasma is tested before release with the Parvo B19 LC PCR Artus test, with a 10.0-UI/μL cutoff. Since this QC procedure was implemented in 2006, not a single batch has been found positive.[7]

Main Characteristics of SD Plasma in France

Comparison with European Pharmacopoeia

Eighteen years after the implementation of the technique, experience has been long enough to show good reproducibility from batch to batch. French requirements for SD plasma differ from the European Pharmacopoeia on the following main points:

- Origin of plasma: Recovered plasma or apheresis plasma in the European Pharmacopoeia; apheresis plasma in the French regulations.

- Protein concentration: >45 g/L in the European Pharmacopoeia; >50 g/L in the French regulations.
- Factor VIII concentration: >0.5 IU/mL in the European Pharmacopoeia; >0.7 IU/mL in the French regulations.

Comparison with Other Licensed Therapeutic Plasmas in France

The best way to provide comparisons between licensed plasmas is to use the data collected by the health authority (ie, the "Agence Française de Sécurité Sanitaire des Produits de Santé," abbreviated AFSSAPS, or the French agency for health safety of health products) during the process of authorization for each type of plasma. As apparent in Table 8-2, SD plasma shows excellent recovery of fibrinogen, Factors V and VIII, protein C, and antithrombin III, while it provides slightly lower (approximately 70%) recovery for protein S and recoveries usually below 50% for $\alpha 2$ antiplasmin and Factor XI. For the latter, it may be a concern in the very rare cases of plasma indication for Factor XI deficiency (as there is at present no available plasma-derived Factor XI concentrate). In order to deal with this potential difficulty, every batch is tested for its Factor XI concentration, and in (the rare) case of a specific indication for a patient being treated for congenital Factor XI deficiency, the blood center is able to select and provide the SD plasma with the highest available Factor XI concentration.

Use of SD Plasma in France

Before 1992, the only therapeutic plasma used was standard fresh frozen plasma. From 1992 to 2006, the licensed therapeutic plasmas were SD plasma and quarantine plasma (ie, the unit of therapeutic plasma being issued after a repeat testing of the corresponding donor is performed following a minimal interval of 4 months). In 2006, the national health authority (Direction Générale de la Santé) declared that all therapeutic plasma should be pathogen-reduced by an authorized method. Apart from SD plasma, two pathogen re-

Table 8-2. Main Characteristics of Therapeutic Plasmas Used in France

Parameters	Unit of Measure	SD Plasma (Range)	MB Plasma	Intercept* Plasma	Quarantine Plasma†
Fibrinogen	g/L	2.7 (2.3-3.6)	2.2 (1.6-3)	2.6 (1.8-4.3)	2.8 (2.3-4.0)
Factor V	% recovery	90 (70-120)	91 (56-130)	87 (57-129)	108 (74-154)
Factor VIII	% recovery	80 (70-100)	93 (53-210)	0.7 (0.4-1.2)‡	107 (55-197)
Factor XI	% recovery	40 (20-50)	76 (54-106)	0.7 (0.5-1)‡	92 (44-125)
Protein C	% recovery	97 (92-107)	108 (77-155)	92 (59-122)	118 (75-175)
Protein S	% recovery	72 (67-79)	107 (73-147)	75 (47-99)	134 (72-200)
Antithrombin III	% recovery	96 (80-105)	105 (95-119)	87 (70-103)	98 (80-112)
$\alpha 2$ antiplasmin	% recovery	39 (37-42)	106 (95-112)	78 (62-94)	105 (88-118)

*Cerus Corporation, Concord, CA.
†Given as a reference.
‡Data given in IU/mL.
SD = solvent/detergent; MB = methylene blue.

duction processes were licensed by the AFSSAPS: the methylene-blue technology developed by Macopharma (Tourcoing, France) and the amotosalen (Intercept) technology developed by Cerus (Concord, CA). These new technologies were introduced in 2007; 2008 was an intermediate year, and in 2009 the shift was completed, after which time quarantine plasma was no longer used.

The use of therapeutic plasma in France has evolved from 1994 to 2008 (see Fig 8-1). Over these 15 years, 2,089,035 quarantine plasma units, 1,812,511 SD plasma units, 20,824 Intercept plasma units (beginning in 2007), and 58,725 methylene-blue plasma units (beginning in 2008) were used. Therefore, SD plasma represents 40% to 50% of therapeutic plasma used in France each year.

Costs

Clearly, the cost of processing SD plasma is much higher than preparing quarantine plasma, and this difference had been taken into account for many years in France in the nationally defined blood component prices. For example, in 2005 the SD plasma price was 66% higher than that of quarantine plasma, representing the approximate difference between the costs of the two manufacturing processes.

This difference in cost led many hospitals to decide, for financial reasons, to use only quarantine plasma. Therefore, in 2006 when the national health authority decided that the use of therapeutic plasma should evolve and progressively shift to 100% pathogen-inactivated components, they simultaneously decided to harmonize the "issuing prices" of the available therapeutic plasmas (ie, SD plasma and quarantine plasma) in order to overcome the reluctance to move to pathogen-reduced components. This national policy was used when two additional pathogen-inactivation processes (methylene blue and Intercept) were introduced in 2007 and 2008. The decision, though logical in terms of public health policy, led to application of an issuing price for plasma units that is slightly below the actual cost of SD plasma. (The difference must be made up through other means.) The detailed issuing prices between 2003 and 2009 are indicated in Fig 8-2.

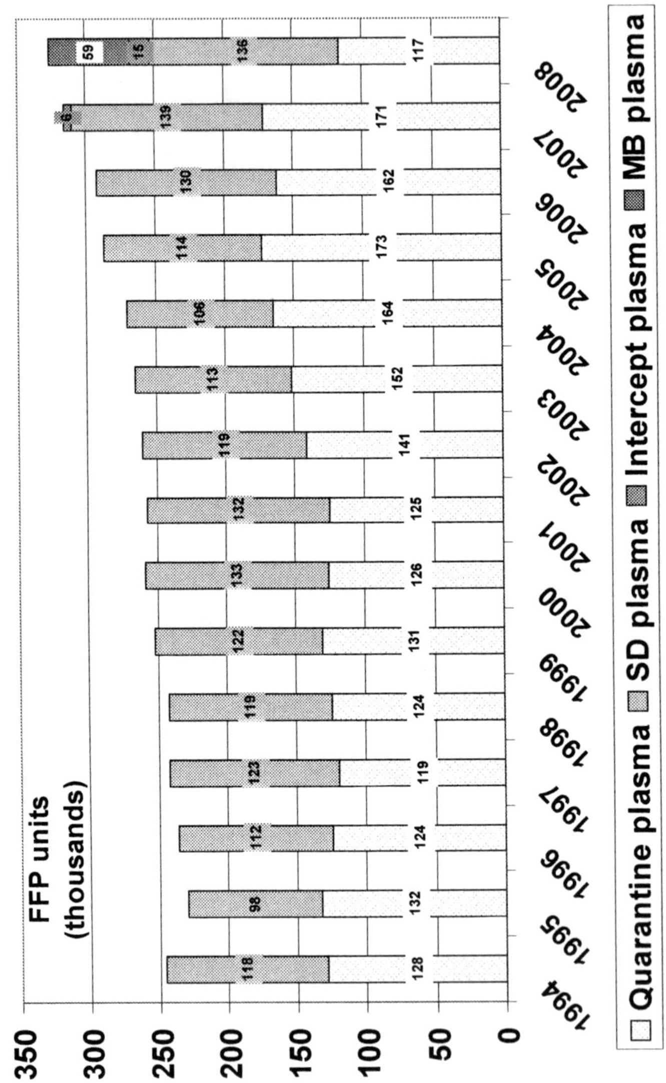

Figure 8-1. Use of therapeutic plasmas in France from 1994 to 2008. Data expressed in thousands of adult therapeutic units (1 adult therapeutic unit = 200 to 250 mL).
FFP = fresh frozen plasma; SD = solvent/detergent; MB = methylene blue.

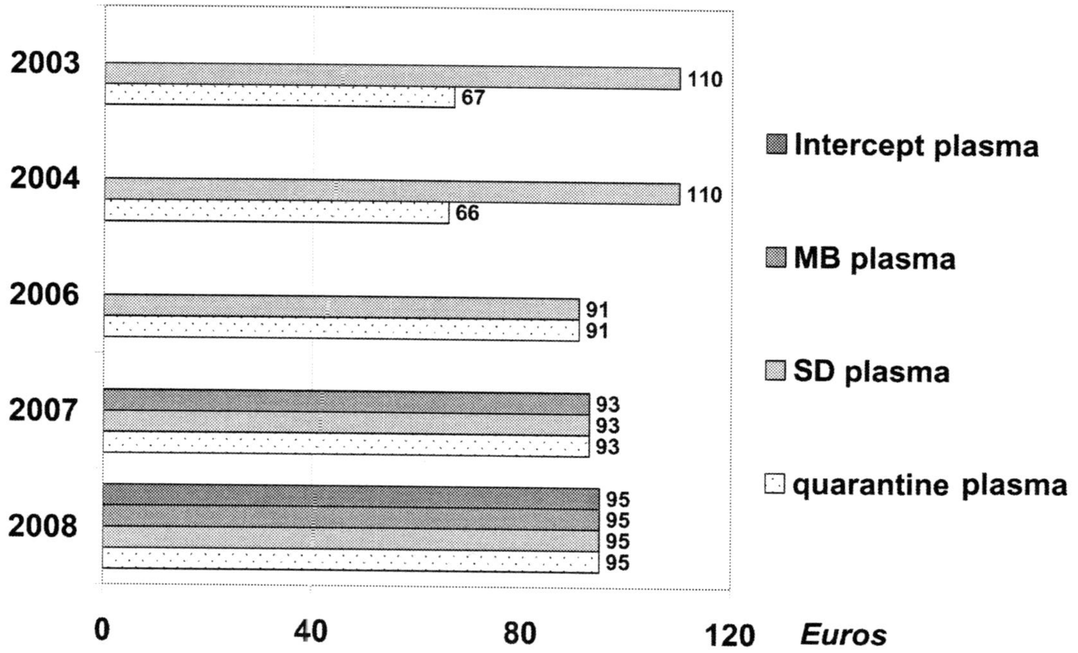

Figure 8-2. Evolution of the nationally defined issuing price in France for therapeutic plasmas from 2003 to 2008 (2005 and 2009 prices were identical to 2004 and 2008, respectively).

Hemovigilance: Surveillance of SD Plasma

Since 1994, a nationwide network of hemovigilance has been in place in France, enabling a dramatic expansion of knowledge concerning adverse reactions to blood components.[11-13] An important piece of information from this system is that plasma transfusion, among all components, least often leads to a recognized reaction and, further, that SD plasma is the blood component with the lowest rate of adverse reactions. In the years 2000 to 2008, the incidence of adverse reactions was 2.6/10,000 SD plasma units, 7/10,000 quarantine plasma units, 18/10,000 red cell concentrate units, 40/10,000 pools of platelet concentrates prepared from whole blood, and 82/10,000 apheresis platelet units.[13]

Specific Adverse Reactions to SD Plasma

Hyperphosphatemia

In the initial manufacturing process of SD plasma, the phosphate concentration was high (mean = 10.3 mmol/L; range = 7.5 to 11.2). This was related to the addition of phosphate during the process (necessary in the SD process to control pH and to optimize Factor VIII recovery) at a relatively high concentration (2.1 g/L). Although this concentration was very much higher than the physiologic one (mean = 0.74 mmol/L, with hyperphosphatemia defined as >1.46 mmol/L), it was considered safe, as phosphates are quickly eliminated by renal excretion. However, in patients with end-stage renal disease, phosphate can accumulate and cause metabolic complications in case of prolonged exposure, as nephrologists know well.[14] Indeed, hyperphosphatemia was observed once in a patient with end-stage renal disease who was then treated by plasma exchange.[15]

Following this observation, it was recommended that phosphate levels be monitored in patients receiving SD plasma and, more particularly, patients likely to develop hyperphosphatemia, such as those with hypoparathyroidism, acromegaly, Paget disease, tumor lysis syndrome, and renal insufficiency. Patients in this latter group would include those presenting with hyperphosphatemia, for whatever reason, and patients receiving high doses of SD plasma, such as those with thrombotic microangiopathy, thrombotic thrombocytopenic purpura, hemolytic-uremic syndrome, and liver transplantation.[16]

In addition, the manufacturing process was revised in order to reduce the phosphate concentrations in the final product. These changes resulted in the phosphate concentration during the treatment being reduced to from 2.1 to 0.69 g/L. This new process led to the present state, where phosphate concentration in SD plasma is 4.81 ±0.41 mmol/L—less than half its value in the initial process. Since this new process was introduced in 2003, no further reports of hyperphosphatemia have been received by the French hemovigilance network.

Enhanced Fibrinolysis After Liver Transplantation

This complication was described in a retrospective study,[17] and the proposed mechanism was the relatively low recovery of α2 antiplasmin in SD plasma. However, these conclusions were not confirmed in other studies in Norway[18] and France,[19] where most liver transplants are performed with SD plasma without such a complication. Indeed, the authors of the retrospective study recognized that their fibrinolysis cases were much more likely to be related to the amount of blood loss.[20]

Other Adverse Reactions

Transfusion-Related Acute Lung Injury

Data from the French hemovigilance network strongly support the assumption that SD plasma does not elicit transfusion-related acute lung injury (TRALI). Table 8-3 indicates the rate of TRALI declared to the network according to the different blood components in the years 2003 to 2008.[13] In that period, TRALI was never found to be related to SD plasma transfusion, while it was considered as related to quarantine plasma in 24 cases. Considering that between 2003 and 2008, 44% of the 1.6 million units of plasma transfused was SD plasma, this difference (0/704,000 vs 24/816,000 units) is highly significant ($p = 3.5 \times 10^{-5}$). In the same period, no case was ob-

Table 8-3. Incidence of TRALI in France, 2003-2008*

Blood Component	TRALI Cases		Units Used	Incidence per Million Units	
	Total	Deaths		Total TRALI	TRALI Deaths
Red cell concentrates (RCC)	60	6	12,461,810	4.8	0.48
Whole-blood-derived platelet concentrates	2	1	1,301,444	8.5	0.77
Apheresis platelet concentrates	41	5	1,118,569	36.7	4.47
Quarantine plasma	24	1	947,264	25.3	1.06
Solvent/detergent plasma	0	0	734,143	0	0
Intercept plasma†	0	0	20,824	0	0
Methylene-blue plasma	0	0	58,525	0	0
Autologous RCC	0	0	217,686	0	0
Total blood components	127	13	16,860,265	7.5	0.77

*Data from the French hemovigilance network.[13]
†Cerus Corporation, Concord, CA.
TRALI = transfusion-related acute lung injury.

served with Intercept or methylene-blue plasmas. However, as only about 20,000 Intercept and 60,000 methylene-blue plasma units were transfused in that period, it is of course not possible to draw firm conclusions about TRALI risk with these components.

Severe Allergic Reactions

In the years 2007 and 2008, several severe allergic reactions were reported with therapeutic plasma, and the incidence per million blood components transfused varied according to the type of therapeutic plasma: 188 for methylene-blue plasma, 96 for Intercept plasma, 74 for quarantine plasma, and 44 for SD plasma.[13] As in the case of TRALI, the lower rate of severe allergic reactions with SD plasma as compared with the other therapeutic plasmas used in France appears statistically significantly lower ($p = 0.004$).

Conclusion

SD plasma technology was implemented in France early after its first development, with later minor modifications to maximize its safety. Parvovirus B19 NAT testing addresses the failure of the SD process to inactivate this nonenveloped virus. The manufacturing of batches from a maximum of 100 donations was introduced to minimize potential dissemination of an infectious agent not detected in blood donors, when the recent emergence of HIV and its unacceptable spread through blood transfusion weighed heavily on the minds of health authorities, transfusionists, prescribers, and the entire society. This policy was reassessed in 2000 when it became clear that the prion responsible for the variant of Creutzfeldt-Jakob disease could be transmitted by blood transfusion. At that time, a risk analysis by health authorities led to the conclusion that the SD-plasma-associated risk was acceptable in France.[21] Since 2000, this risk analysis has been re-assessed several times, with the same conclusion regarding the use of SD plasma.[22]

Apart from the clear absence of relationship between TRALI and SD plasma, hemovigilance data provide good evidence that specific adverse reactions to SD plasma occur very infrequently, with only one case of hyperphosphatemia and no excess of fibrinolysis among liver transplant patients. Moreover, the rate of adverse reactions to SD plasma is by far the lowest among all blood components, including other therapeutic plasmas. However, with respect to the therapeutic plasma supply, the French consider the use of several sources as the best way to avoid shortage in case of process and/or provider failure. Therefore, SD, Intercept, and methylene-blue plasmas are used, the former representing 40% to 50% of the overall supply.

References

1. Horowitz B, Wiebe ME, Lippin A, Stryker MH. Inactivation of viruses in labile blood derivatives. I. Disruption of lipid-enveloped viruses by tri(n-butyl) phosphate detergent combinations. Transfusion 1985;25:516-22.
2. Prince AM, Horowitz B, Brotman B. Sterilization of hepatitis and HTLV-III viruses by exposure to tri(n-butyl)phosphate and sodium cholate. Lancet 1986;1:706-10.
3. Piet MPJ, Chin S, Prince AM, et al. The use of tri(n-butyl)phosphate (TNBP) detergent mixtures to inactivate hepatitis viruses and human immunodeficiency virus in plasma and its subsequent fractionation. Transfusion 1990; 30:591-8.
4. Horowitz B, Bonomo R, Prince AM, et al. Solvent/detergent-treated plasma: A virus-inactivated substitute for fresh frozen plasma. Blood 1992;79:826-31.
5. Hellstern P, Sachse H, Schwinn H, Oberfrank K. Manufacture and in vitro characterization of a solvent/detergent-treated human plasma. Vox Sang 1992;63:178-85.
6. Piquet Y, Janvier G, Selosse P, et al. Virus inactivation of fresh frozen plasma by a solvent detergent procedure: Biological results. Vox Sang 1992;63:251-6.
7. Petermann R, Piquet Y, Pinteus J, et al. Détection du génome viral du parvovirus B19 dans les pools de plasmas servant à la préparation du plasma frais congelé traité pour viroattenuation par solvant détergent (PVASD): Expérience de l'AFSSAPS et de l'EFS Aquitaine-Limousin (EFS AL). Saint Denis, France: AFFSAPS, 2008. [Available at http://www.afssaps.fr/var/afssaps_site/storage/original/application/d06b665c1e4ea96689ac3783e16a832e.pdf (accessed May 8, 2010.)]
8. Jeanne M, Piquet Y, Ivanovic Z, et al. Variations of Factor VIII:C plasma levels with respect to the blood group ABO. Transfus Med 2004;2:187-8.
9. Kao KJ, Scornik J, Small SJ. Enzyme-linked immunoassay for anti-HLA antibodies: An alternative to panel studies by lymphocytotoxicity. Transplantation 1993;55:192-6.
10. Jiang AF, Lalezari P. A micro-technique for detection of leukocyte agglutinins. J Immunol Methods 1975;7:103-8.

11. Andreu G, Morel P, Forestier F, et al. Haemovigilance network in France: Organization and analysis of immediate transfusion incident reports from 1994 to 1998. Transfusion 2002;42:1356-64.
12. Rebibo D, Hauser L, Slimani A, et al. The French haemovigilance system: Organization and results for 2003. Transfus Apher Sci 2004;31:145-53.
13. Agence Française de Sécurité Sanitaire des Produits de Santé. Rapport annuel hémovigilance 2008. Saint Denis, France: AFSSAPS, 2009. [Available at http://www.afssaps.fr/Activites/Hemovigilance/Hemovigilance/(offset)/0 (rapport Activité Hémovigilance 28/07/2009; accessed May 8, 2010).]
14. Ritz E. The clinical management of hyperphosphatemia. J Nephrol 2005; 18:221-8.
15. Thiéry G, Jacobs F, Bussel A, et al. Acute hyperphosphatemia after plasma exchange with S/D-treated plasma. Transfusion 2004;44:947-8.
16. Agence Française de Sécurité Sanitaire des Produits de Santé. [Transfusion of fresh frozen plasma: Products, indications.] (Recommendations; August 2002) Saint Denis, France: AFSSAPS, 2002. [Available at http://www.afssaps.fr/var/afssaps_site/storage/original/application/f21a8be3650653cabb6391cf7845226f.pdf (accessed May 8, 2010).]
17. de Jonge J, Groenland TH, Metselaar HJ, et al. Fibrinolysis during liver transplantation is enhanced by using solvent/detergent virus-inactivated plasma (ESDEP). Anesth Analg 2002;94:1127-31.
18. Solheim BG, Bergan A, Brosstad F, et al. Fibrinolysis during liver transplant and use of solvent/detergent virus-inactivated plasma (ESDEP/Octaplas). Anesth Analg 2003;96:1230-1.
19. Ozier Y, Rieux C. Liver transplantation, solvent-detergent treated plasma and antifibrinolytics. Anesth Analg 2003;96:1231.
20. de Jonge J, Groenland TH, Metselaar HJ, et al. Fibrinolysis during liver transplantation is enhanced by using solvent/detergent virus-inactivated plasma (ESDEP) (letter). Anesth Analg 2003;96:1231.
21. Agence Française de Sécurité Sanitaire des Produits de Santé. Analyse du risque de transmission de la nouvelle variante de la maladie de Creutzfeldt Jakob par le sang et ses dérivés. (Recommendations; December 11, 2000) Saint Denis, France: AFSSAPS, 2000. [Available at http://www.afssaps.fr/var/afssaps_site/storage/original/application/32cc7caa1bdbc83f7d36dfd01e0ee4ef.pdf (accessed May 8, 2010).]
22. Agence Française de Sécurité Sanitaire des Produits de Santé. Analyse du risque de transmission de la variant de la maladie de Creutzfeldt Jakob (vMCJ) et de la forme sporadique de la maladie de Creutzfeldt-Jakob par les produits de santé d'origine humaine. (November 2007 report) Saint Denis, France: AFSSAPS, 2007. [Available at http://www.afssaps.fr/var/afssaps_site/storage/original/application/a2c27cf0f2791315d7f50bdbcc04d82c.pdf (accessed May 8, 2010).

In: AuBuchon JP, Prowse CV, eds.
Pathogen Inactivation: The Penultimate Paradigm Shift
Bethesda, MD: AABB Press, 2010

9

Ireland: Imported US-Source Solvent/Detergent Plasma

WILLIAM G. MURPHY, MD, FRCPEDIN, FRCPATH, AND OLGA MIKULICH, MD, PHD, MRCPI*

IN 2002 THE IRISH BLOOD TRANSFUSION SERVICE (IBTS) replaced almost all of its fresh frozen plasma (FFP) for clinical use with solvent/detergent (SD) plasma from volunteer US donors. This was part of a systematic response to the threat of variant Creutzfeldt-Jakob disease (vCJD) from blood transfusion. The logic governing the decision was that it was possible, to an unknowable extent, that vCJD could be transmitted by transfusion of blood and blood components, and that Ireland was at a considerable, if unquantifiable,

---

William G. Murphy, MD, FRCPEdin, FRCPath, Medical and Scientific Director, Irish Blood Transfusion Service, National Blood Centre, and Clinical Senior Lecturer, School of Medicine and Medical Science, University College, Dublin, and Olga Mikulich, MD, PhD, MRCPI,* Specialist Registrar, Department of Medicine, St James's Hospital, Dublin, Ireland
*Formerly Dr V. Chekrizova.

The authors have disclosed no conflicts of interest.

risk of having presymptomatic and infectious blood donors in its population. Although this risk was unlikely to be as high as that in the United Kingdom, it was nonetheless possible that it was on a similar order of magnitude. It was therefore reasonable to conclude that avoiding use of plasma from Irish blood donors might reduce the risk to patients needing transfusion.

How big was that risk? Attempts at quantifying it always left considerable room for doubt.[1,2] The possible, though perhaps not probable, consequences of getting the decision wrong were the more cogent issues, at least to the IBTS. If it turns out that there will be very few transmissions of vCJD from Irish plasma, or even none at all, then the downside, at the very worst, would be that €2.5 million was spent per year, from a total health-care budget of €17 billion (ie, 15 thousandths of a percent) for no calculable gain. If, on the other hand, even one donor among the 100,000 who donate yearly were to have transmitted vCJD through plasma—well within the calculated tolerances for the prevalence in Ireland based on extrapolations from UK studies and estimates—then the decision would have averted a human tragedy at a price that the Irish State and public would, at least in 2002, have been happy to pay. The IBTS consciously managed a real and quantifiable threat rather than prevaricated over an unquantifiable risk.

How does one manage an unknowable risk? How does one deal with issues of life and death that could involve many people when those issues are surrounded by uncertainty? In fact, managing complexity and complex risks and threats is part of everyday life, for example, when people obtain home insurance and face fire risks, travel risks, and even risks involved in getting home at night. Several tactics are employed throughout life in an almost intuitive way, consistently and deliberately, even if not always knowingly.

Managing Threats Instead of Risks

A risk is generally quantifiable—there is a mathematical expression with a one above the line and a number below the line; from this it can be known that, on average, exposure to a particular phenomenon or action a given number of times will likely result in a misadventure, or that the incidence of that misadventure is predictable in a population exposed to the phenomenon or action. The risk of misadventure may be avoided or diminished by moving to a different population or by reducing the frequency of exposure to the phenomenon, but the risk remains the same for that population. Threats are less quantifiable in numeric terms—they may be near or remote; they may be large or small. Actions taken to address threats depend on their proximity and size. The Cold War, for example, was waged largely by threat, whether real or imagined, and threat management. Threat management is also applied to tsunamis and earthquakes.

The key features of successful threat management[3] can be inferred from sources outside of clinical medicine and public health, such as natural history, engineering, military practice, construction, seismology, and sociology. These features include surveillance and assessment of size and proximity, avoidance and evasion, layered defenses, damage limitation (containment, cellularity, repair, and redundancy), and contingency (including escape). As a whole, these confer robustness and resilience, and each feature provides an independent quantum of resistance to threat (see Table 9-1).

The steps that the IBTS took to address the threat of vCJD transmission from blood transfusion in Ireland were taken within the framework of threat management (see Table 9-2): The risk of transmitting vCJD from transfusion of Irish plasma was unknown, and there was very little that could be done to reduce that underlying risk. Consequently, the action taken was to reduce the exposure of patients in Ireland to that risk, by replacing plasma from Irish blood donors with plasma from an area likely to have a much lower level of vCJD in its donors.

Surveillance and Assessment of Size and Proximity

The purpose of surveillance and assessment activities was to maintain a constant awareness of emerging data on the nature of the illness, its extent, and the behavior of the agent, and to do this in a consistent, formal, and properly resourced manner. Activities consisted mainly of constant networking with experts in the field to ensure early warning of emerging information, as well as frequent reviews of what was known and what was being done about it. A large amount of effort went into this: local conferences with invited experts, commissioned reports, and attendance by one or two designated individuals at all or almost all significant scientific meetings

Table 9-1. The Elements of Threat Management

Element	Properties (Example)	Measurement (Example)	Actions
Assessment of threat	Existence (Could BSE be transmitted by blood transfusion?)	Binary (yes or no)	Constant surveillance
	Proximity (Is there a problem with BSE and blood transfusion now?)	Semiquantitative (near, imminent, remote, unknown)	High-grade information/intelligence inflow
	Magnitude (If so, how big could it be?)	Semiquantitative assessment of potential for damage	Continual updating and assessment of plans in the light of incoming information
Avoidance/evasion	Finding an alternative route or source of supply, or removing exposure to the threat (eg, avoidance of blood use)	Qualitative: identify the available tactics and strategies	Assess the feasibility and costs of alternatives
Defense	Layered defenses: several different, complimentary, and preferably unlinked and independent (or, better, autonomous) parts (testing, donor exclusions, filtration, leukocyte reduction)	Qualitative: identify the available tactics and strategies	Ensure all effective or potentially effective actions/elements are known and understood, and, where adopted, implemented and functional

Damage limitation	Detection of incursion/ failure of defenses: containment and cellularity within the blood supply, repair of defenses, backup for critical component failures, creation of inbuilt redundancy	Qualitative: identify the available or potential tactics and strategies	Implement capability, test and maintain functionality, build in redundancy where possible
Contingency: system-wide critical failure	Developing plans with other blood services unlikely to be affected, for support in the event of critical failure of supply; alternatives [cancellation of elective surgery within the State and sending children abroad for surgery (equivalent to escape and survival at individual level)]	Qualitative: identify the available tactics and strategies	As above (equivalent to checking the life jackets on aircraft or in the life rafts on cruise ships)

BSE = bovine spongiform encephalopathy.

Table 9-2. Threat Management and vCJD: The IBTS Response

Element of Threat Management	Actions Taken
Assessment of threat (surveillance)	• Local conferences with invited experts • Commissioned report • Attendance by one or two designated individuals at significant scientific meetings in Europe and the USA Constant survey of the scientific literature Early engagement with manufacturers of emerging detection and removal technologies Formal reviews twice monthly
Avoidance/ evasion	Implementation of alternatives to transfusion of blood components from Irish, UK, or other European risk-area donors: • Exclusive use of recombinant Factor VIII and Factor IX beginning in 1997 • Use of US plasma as preferred source for nonrecombinant factor concentrates distributed by the IBTS • Replacement of almost all plasma for clinical use with US-sourced solvent/detergent plasma • Replacement of almost all cryoprecipitate for clinical use with fibrinogen concentrate from US-sourced plasma
Defense	Exclusion of donors with increased risk through UK residence Leukocyte depletion of all fresh blood components Phase I clinical trials of prion-filtered red cells (test likely to be implemented as soon as available)
Damage limitation	Exclusion of previously transfused persons from donation
Contingency	No formal contingency system was enacted, though, particularly in the earlier years, a number of contingency plans were seriously considered, including sending children abroad for elective surgery and collecting blood for Irish use in purpose-specific collection programs abroad in collaboration with other national blood services (eg, organizing collections in geographic areas not fully used by self-sufficient blood services in countries with a large Irish diaspora)

vCJD: variant Creutzfeldt-Jakob disease; IBTS = Irish Blood Transfusion Service.

in Europe and the United States; constant survey of the scientific literature; and early engagement with the manufacturers of emerging technologies for testing and removal. Formal reviews took place twice monthly: at internal medical department meetings and at meetings of the medical subcommittee of the Board of Governance, a body that included non-transfusion-service senior clinicians.

Avoidance and Evasion

Donors were deferred who had increased exposure to vCJD as a result of prior residence in the United Kingdom. The effect of this on blood safety was limited because of the very large degree of exposure of people within Ireland to bovine spongiform encephalopathy (BSE)-infected indigenous and UK-sourced beef.[1] Avoidance also included sourcing plasma from outside the BSE-risk zone and, later on, replacing cryoprecipitate use with use of fibrinogen concentrate from US donors. In Ireland, plasma-derived Factor VIII and Factor IX concentrates had been discontinued in 1997 and replaced with recombinant factors. In addition, blood collection was discontinued from people who had been transfused either ever outside of Ireland or since 1980 within Ireland. This closed a feedback loop—after 2001 the most likely source of infection from vCJD in Ireland may well have been from transfusion; preventing people who had been exposed to this source from passing on infection by the same route reduced the risk to others.

Avoiding unnecessary transfusions of red cells, platelets, and plasma probably constitutes the most readily available method of evading the threat of vCJD infection at the individual patient level: Ireland's usage of red cells is low compared to other developed nations (34 units per 1000 population annually, compared to the 38.1 per 1000 annual average for developed countries, as reported to the World Health Organization).[4] However, platelet usage per capita at 5.5 per 1000 population is high compared to other European countries, although similar to the rate of 5.9 per 1000 population in the United States (2001 US data).[5]

Defenses

Defenses from infectious donors in the pool are limited. Universal leukocyte reduction was introduced in 1999 on the basis of some evidence that suggested it might reduce infectivity.[6,7] Early trials of vCJD filters for red cells were conducted, but funding has not yet allowed broad adoption of them.[8,9]

Damage Limitation

Containment and cellularity are related but different aspects of coping with a threat that has breached defenses. Ensuring that people cannot donate if they may have been exposed to infection from transfusion is one form of containment; cellularity is difficult to achieve but can be addressed by "buddying" donors and recipients for transfusion-dependent donors and, where possible, reducing both recipient-to-donor exposure and donor-to-recipient exposure. This last point merited serious deliberation. Although using apheresis platelets substantially reduces the risk to the individual patient receiving the transfusion, it requires that apheresis donors donate much more frequently than whole blood donors to meet the demand for platelets. Each plateletpheresis donor donates up to 12 times a year, with a mean number of four donations. Each apheresis donation goes to a median of two patients, similar to a whole blood donation divided into red cell and platelet components. If an infectious donor is undetected in the apheresis donor pool, a mean of 40 and a maximum of over 100 recipients could be infected for a window period of 5 years. With an infectious whole blood donor, the mean number of recipients over the same period is 16, and the maximum is 40. Ireland has approximately 50 times more whole blood donors than apheresis donors. Therefore, the possibility of a major outbreak of 40 or more infections was traded for the much higher possibility of a limited outbreak exposing much fewer individuals. However, because the risk to the individual patient is always lower the fewer donors they are exposed to (provided the donor demography is similar), that is the preferred option from the recipient's point of view.[10]

The Decision to Use Solvent/Detergent Plasma

Before the vCJD problem came to dominate concerns over blood safety, it had become generally recognized that FFP could be subjected to further safety measures beyond the steps already in use—ie, donor selection and virology testing. Additional steps such as placement in quarantine and treatment with methylene blue, solvent/detergent, or amotosalen added a further degree of safety against window-period transmissions of tested viruses and (apart from quarantine) a degree of safety against emerging viruses and other infectious agents.

After an initial assessment of methylene blue for individual units, investigators experienced regulatory concerns over source materials and were unhappy with the loss of Factor VIII and fibrinogen across the process, at least in the Irish experience. Amotosalen treatment was being considered and a small-scale quarantine program had begun when the decision was made in 2000-2001 to seek a source of plasma outside of the BSE-risk zone, following a review of available options and actions after the publication of the sheep transmission data in 2000.[11] It was determined that US blood services were the most feasible source of sufficient volumes of plasma for clinical use at that time. A number of European services could have supplied Ireland, but there was likely to be a lower risk from the United States than from any European country. In retrospect, a Scandinavian source for the plasma might have been adequate—the risk was likely to be low and would have been relatively improved by use of a nonpooled product compared to a pooled one. However, the Scandinavians were not contemplating nucleic acid testing of donations at that time, which would have mandated a pathogen-reduction step for Irish purposes. Sources outside of the United States and Europe, such as Canada, New Zealand, Australia, or Japan, were not considered to offer any real advantage and brought additional logistic problems. Ultimately, pathogen-inactivated plasma from noncommercial US blood donors was deemed to offer the best solution to the problem of obtaining plasma for clinical use from a low vCJD and other infectious-disease risk source.

Initially, individual US donor units treated with amotosalen were assessed. Losses of Factor VIII activity were unacceptably high because of the need to ship the plasma frozen and then thaw, treat, and refreeze it. Attempts to arrange for the plasma to be treated at the source blood center before thawing were thwarted by regulatory obstacles on both sides of the Atlantic. SD plasma in pools of 1700 donors provided an acceptable degree of safety over single-donor Irish plasma, as the risk of vCJD in US donors was considered negligible for the purposes of pooled plasma products. Although surveillance for BSE in the US herd was not comparable to that in place in

Ireland, the possible exposure of US donors to dietary vCJD risk was many orders of magnitude below that of Irish donors.

There were other advantages: apart from protection from window-period infections, SD plasma at that time was emerging as having low to zero risk of transfusion-related acute lung injury (TRALI); over 2,000,000 doses had been transfused without a single pharmacovigilance report either of TRALI or of infectious disease transmission. In addition, unit activity was more predictable, and dosage was more sensible—every bag contained the same volume of plasma.

Finally, the introduction of a new pharmaceutical approach to plasma transfusion presented an opportunity for a national program of education in plasma transfusion and, in particular, in optimal management of warfarin toxicity, a major and generally inappropriate indication for plasma usage.

It is important to stress, however, that the decision to use Octapharma's SD plasma over the Cerus amotosalen-treated product was ultimately based on logistic rather than safety grounds. It is not inconceivable that at some stage in the future Ireland may switch to a single-donor product, though recent developments in prion-removal technology for pooled SD plasma may confer an additional level of safety on that product.[12]

All plasma for the program comes from a single US blood center—the South Texas Blood and Tissue Center. It is shipped at Ireland's expense to Vienna, Austria, where it is manufactured in requested batches into Octaplas [(Octapharma AG, Lachen, Switzerland) ie, group-specific, SD virus-inactivated plasma in pools of approximately 1700 donations] or Uniplas (Octapharma), an unlicensed product made from pools of plasma of different groups in a process identical to Octaplas, with very low residual titers of anti-A or anti-B. Uniplas is intended to function as universal plasma that can be transfused to all patients regardless of their blood group.[13] In Ireland, it is used almost exclusively for type AB patients as a pragmatic solution to the problem of not being able to collect enough AB plasma for a group-specific batch from the single supplying US center.

Costs

Octaplas from recovered US plasma incurred a considerable increment in cost over indigenous recovered FFP. In the first place, indigenous FFP is a marginal product, and any true expense incurred to the health service budget was minimal. Second, US FFP has to be paid for with funds that leave the country; shipping and Octaplas manufacturing are also real costs with cash outflow from the health service and the national purse. Ultimately the net cost to the exchequer is over ∈2,000,000.00 per year.

The Changeover Process

The changeover was relatively easy: Ireland is a small country of approximately 4 million inhabitants with fewer than 40 hematologists and only 10 large teaching hospitals (although there are a further 51 hospital blood banks in smaller hospitals). There is only one blood service, operating from two blood centers. All liver transplantation is performed in one hospital, and there are only a handful of cardiac surgery units, only one of which treats children.

Approximately 25,000 units of plasma are transfused annually (along with 135,000 red cell units and, at that time, 16,000 units of platelets). Over a period of a few weeks, a hematologist from the IBTS visited all major hospitals and most of the smaller ones to introduce the program and product. Over a matter of days, the new product was shipped to hospitals throughout the country, and the stocks of FFP were returned to the IBTS for destruction.

There was general acceptance of the measure, and initial feedback was favorable. A large survey was conducted of all the units used in pediatric and adult patients with liver disease and in all neonatal cases, along with all transfusions in obstetric and gynecologic emergencies over the first 18 months of use in three large hospitals in Dublin from April 1, 2002 (when SD plasma was introduced) through October 31, 2003.[14] Forty-one neonates received 67 transfusions of SD plasma at a mean dose (± standard deviation) of 18.4 ±13.2 mL/kg^{-1}. Thirty-one (75.6%) patients had coagulopathy without hemorrhage (either disseminated intravascular coagulopathy or other coagulopathy); a further eight (19.5%) had clinical hemorrhage (excluding intraventricular hemorrhage) that complicated a coagulopathy. Thirty-eight obstetric and gynecologic patients received 57 SD plasma transfusions at a mean dose of 15.3 ±7.7 mL/kg^{-1}. Thirty-six women (94.7%) had hemorrhage, with a mean blood loss per patient of 3345.8 ±2738.1 mL. Fifteen children with liver disease received 33 SD plasma transfusions at a mean volume of

38.0 ±41.5 mL/kg^{-1} body weight. Seventeen adult patients with severe end-stage liver disease were transfused with SD plasma either following liver transplantation or before other invasive procedures, at a mean dose of 10.2 ±3.4 mL/kg^{-1}. There were statistically significant decreases in mean activated partial thromboplastin time and prothrombin time in neonates, in obstetric and gynecologic patients, and in patients with liver disease. Complete correction of coagulation parameters was not achieved in any case in the liver transplant group. No adverse reactions were observed for SD plasma infusion. Use of SD plasma in these groups appeared safe and improved laboratory indices of coagulopathy.

The liver transplantation unit, however, reported two cases of death associated with severe coagulopathy, excessive bleeding, fibrinolysis, and refractory hemodynamic instability among the first 22 cases after the changeover to Octaplas.[15] This was unexpected considering recent experience and caused the unit to suspend the use of SD plasma and restore the use of FFP for intraoperative use in liver transplantation; this situation persists to date. Loss of antiplasmin activity in the preparation of Octaplas was considered a likely contributor.[16,17] The authors made the point that data between countries are not strictly comparable because the methods of preparation of the starting plasma may differ; in this case, plasma for Octaplas manufacturing may not be frozen until the day after collection, unlike the Norwegian material, which is frozen for shipping to Vienna within 8 hours of collection. Thus, notwithstanding the considerable favorable experience in Norway, where SD plasma had been used in over 200 consecutive liver transplants without problems[18]—and in a relatively small prospective randomized study in the United Kingdom[17] involving 49 patients with severe liver disease, including 25 undergoing liver transplantation, where adverse effects of SD plasma compared to FFP were not observed—the current view remains that the balance of risk favors FFP in patients undergoing liver transplantation in Ireland. The prospect of switching to the prion-filtered product, which has a higher content of antiplasmin than Octaplas, provides an opportunity to revisit this issue in the near future.

The annual rate of clinical use of plasma showed very little change after the introduction of SD plasma, remaining between 23,000 and 25,000 units issued per year. It is possible that several countervailing trends resulted in this apparent stability; however, the requirement for a degree of speed to replace FFP with SD plasma prevented a useful before-and-after study at the time. Warfarin reversal was largely treated by FFP infusions before the introduction of Octaplas, but at the changeover clinicians were asked to review this practice in the light of current guidelines. This led to a rise in the use of concentrates of Factors II, VII, IX, and X in Ireland. The associated, expected reduction in the use of plasma may have been offset by an increase in the mean dose infused per treatment episode from a standard 2-unit transfusion of FFP to a per-kilogram dose for SD plasma.

Cryoprecipitate

Like much of the English-speaking part of the world and in contrast to much of the rest of it, Ireland used cryoprecipitate made from FFP as a source of fibrinogen in the treatment of acquired hypofibrinogenemia, especially in obstetric bleeding. Usage was about 10% that of FFP. After the replacement of FFP, several options were considered and abandoned, including the manufacture of cryoprecipitate from SD plasma and from amotosalen-treated plasma either made abroad or from imported, treated plasma. In 2009, based on recent studies that had indicated equivalence between cryoprecipitate and fibrinogen concentrate in clinical practice,[19,20] and in the light of extensive experience with fibrinogen concentrate in other countries (notwithstanding the absence of good comparative or even observational clinical study data), the IBTS opted to replace cryoprecipitate with fibrinogen concentrate made exclusively from US plasma donors. This process has been completed, with the exception of neonatal cardiac surgery, where further consideration and analysis are required before replacement of the profound uncertainty of vCJD risk with a change in this critical and currently stable area of surgical hemostasis.

References

1. Harney MS, Ghani AC, Donnelly CA, et al. vCJD risk in the Republic of Ireland. BMC Infect Dis 2003;3:28.

2. Ghani AC, Ferguson NM, Donnelly CA, Anderson RM. Predicted vCJD mortality in Great Britain. Nature 2000;406(6796):583-4.
3. Murphy W. Managing threats rather than risks in blood transfusion: Robust design for a complex system. Transfusion 2006;46:2011-13.
4. World Health Organization. WHO global database on blood safety (GDBS) and blood safety indicators. Geneva: WHO, 2009. [Summary data available from Fact sheet no. 279 (November 2009) at www.who.int/mediacentre/factsheets/fs279/en/index.html (accessed May 10, 2010).]
5. Sullivan MT, Cotten R, Read EJ, Wallace EL. Blood collection and transfusion in the United States in 2001. Transfusion 2007;47:385-94.
6. Klein MA, Frigg R, Flechsig E, et al. A crucial role for B cells in neuroinvasive scrapie. Nature 1997;390:687-90.
7. Murphy W. International views on universal leucodepletion: The perspective in NBS, Ireland. Transfus Sci 1998;19:349-50.
8. Murphy CV, Eakins E, Fagan J, et al. In vitro assessment of red-cell concentrates in SAG-M filtered through the MacoPharma P-CAPT prion-reduction filter. Transfus Med 2009;19:109-16.
9. Cahill MR, Murphy T, Khan M, et al. Phase I/II safety study of transfusion of prion-filtered red cell concentrates in transfusion-dependent patients. Vox Sang 2010 Mar 22 (epub ahead of print).
10. Dobra SA, Bennett PG. vCJD and blood transfusion: Risk assessment in the United Kingdom. Transfus Clin Biol 2006;13:307-11.
11. Houston F, Foster JD, Chong A, et al. Transmission of BSE by blood transfusion in sheep. Lancet 2000;356:999-1000.
12. Neisser-Svae A, Bailey A, Gregori L, et al. Prion removal effect of a specific affinity ligand introduced into the manufacturing process of the pharmaceutical quality solvent/detergent (S/D)-treated plasma OctaplasLG. Vox Sang 2009;97:226-33.
13. Noddeland H, Töllöfsrud S, Svennevig J, et al. Universal solvent/detergent-treated fresh frozen plasma (Uniplas)—rationale and clinical properties. Thromb Res 2002;107(Suppl 1):S33-7.
14. Chekrizova V, Murphy WG. Solvent-detergent plasma: Use in neonatal patients, in adult and paediatric patients with liver disease and in obstetric and gynaecological emergencies. Transfus Med 2006;16:85-91.
15. Magner JJ, Crowley KJ, Boylan JF. Fatal fibrinolysis during orthotopic liver transplantation in patients receiving solvent/detergent-treated plasma (Octaplas). J Cardiothorac Vasc Anaesth 2007;21:410-13.
16. Mast AE, Stadanlick JE, Lockett JM, Dietzen DJ. Solvent/detergent-treated plasma has decreased antitrypsin activity and absent antiplasmin activity. Blood 1999;94:3922-7.
17. de Jonge J, Groenland TH, Metselaar HJ, et al. Fibrinolysis during liver transplantation is enhanced by using solvent/detergent virus-inactivated plasma (ESDEP). Anesth Analg 2002;94:1127-31.
18. Solheim BG, Bergan A, Brosstad F, et al. Fibrinolysis during liver transplant and use of solvent/detergent virus-inactivated plasma (ESDEP/Octaplas). Anesth Analg 2003;96:1230-1.

19. Danés AF, Cuenca LG, Bueno SR, et al. Efficacy and tolerability of human fibrinogen concentrate administration to patients with acquired fibrinogen deficiency and active or in high-risk severe bleeding. Vox Sang 2008;94:221-6.
20. Weinkove R, Rangarajan S. Fibrinogen concentrate for acquired hypofibrinogenaemic states. Transfus Med 2008;18:151-7.

In: AuBuchon JP, Prowse CV, eds.
Pathogen Inactivation: The Penultimate Paradigm Shift
Bethesda, MD: AABB Press, 2010

10

United Kingdom: Imported US-Source Methylene-Blue-Treated Plasma

CHRISTOPHER V. PROWSE, DPHIL, FRCPATH

IN THE UNITED KINGDOM (UK), CONCERNS OVER variant Creutzfeldt-Jakob disease (vCJD) have been the chief driver for the types of plasma in use, although methylene-blue-treated plasma (MB plasma) was first introduced as a result of concerns relating to the viral safety of plasma. Similar concerns led to the fairly widespread adoption of "safer" plasmas around Europe. Currently, plasma for children in the UK is sourced from donors in the United States and is treated with methylene blue after importation to ad-

---

Christopher V. Prowse, DPhil, FRCPath, Research Director, Scottish National Blood Transfusion Service, Edinburgh, Scotland, United Kingdom

The author has disclosed financial relationships with Baxter, CaridianBCT, and MacoPharma.

dress any differences in pathogen prevalence or testing regimes between the two countries. For patients who may receive large volumes of plasma (those requiring large-volume plasma exchanges or who have a coagulation deficiency for which no protein concentrate is available—chiefly patients with thrombotic thrombocytopenic purpura, or TTP), the recommendation is to use pooled solvent/detergent-treated plasma. All other patients who are prescribed plasma receive fresh frozen plasma (FFP) from standard UK donors. The characteristics of the products used and some of the alternatives now available are summarized in Table 10-1. Cryoprecipitate is also provided from both UK and imported MB plasma. Recently a recommendation has been made that all UK patients should receive plasma that has been imported and/or treated to further reduce any risk of vCJD transmission.[1]

The first publication regarding a technology for the pathogen inactivation of whole plasma was in 1991 from the Springe Group, near Hannover, Germany, describing the use of methylene-blue photo-inactivation.[2-4] This was soon followed by the development of solvent/detergent-treated plasma (SD plasma) in 1992 and subsequently by other technologies.[5] At that time there were still serious concerns about the infectivity of blood in the wake of descriptions of the human immunodeficiency virus and the hepatitis C virus. As a result, many European countries adopted regulations that required the use of "virus-safe" plasma. MB plasma was widely used in Germany, Switzerland, and Austria, while SD plasma was used in many US centers during the early 1990s.[6] At that time most MB plasma was produced at the Springe Red Cross Blood Centre from single donations of frozen-thawed plasma, to which a metered dose of methylene blue was added before photo-inactivation. That process is still used and has been adopted by the Grifols company in Spain. In collaboration with Springe, Baxter [Deerfield, IL (PathInact)], and subsequently MacoPharma [Tourcoing, France (Macotronic)], developed equipment for methylene-blue treatment of plasma in blood banks (see Chapter 5).

Introduction of Virus-Safe Plasma in the UK

In the face of concerns about the viral safety of transfusion, the Scottish National Blood Transfusion Service (SNBTS) undertook an op-

Table 10-1. Fresh Plasma Products Used in the UK and Alternatives

Product	Use in UK	Company	CE Marking	Mechanism of Virus Inactivation	Comments
Standard fresh frozen plasma	All patients over 16 unless high-volume users	Not applicable	Not applicable	Not applicable	Recent recommendation: all plasma should be imported[1]
OctaPlas (solvent/detergent-treated pooled plasma)	Recommended for large-volume plasma exchange (eg, in TTP) to reduce vCJD risk	OctaPharma AG (Lachen, Switzerland)	1998 UK product license (by Medicines and Healthcare Products Regulatory Agency as medicine)	Chemical disruption of lipid envelope (plasma is also screened for hepatitis A virus and parvovirus B19)	• Reduced risk of TRALI • Potential to share any infection among multiple vials • Prion-reduced product under assessment (OctaPlas LG) • Low protein S and antiplasmin

(Continued)

Table 10-1. Fresh Plasma Products Used in the UK and Alternatives (Continued)

Product	Use in UK	Company	CE Marking	Mechanism of Virus Inactivation	Comments
Theraflex (methylene blue + visible light)	Patients under 16 to reduce vCJD risk	MacoPharma (Tourcoing, France)	2001	Photodynamic	• Plasma imported from USA • Reduced vCJD and virus risk
Intercept (amotosalen + UVA)	Not at present	Cerus (Concord, CA)	2006	Photochemical	Reduced virus risk
Mirasol (riboflavin + UVA/UVB)	Not at present	CaridianBCT (Lakewood, CO)	2008	Photochemical	Reduced virus risk
Quarantine plasma	Not at present	Not applicable	Not applicable	Rescreen donor ≥3 months before using unit	Addresses only pathogens for which screening is in place

CE = Conformité Européenne; UVA = ultraviolet A (light); UVB = ultraviolet B (light); TTP = thrombotic thrombocytopenic purpura; vCJD = variant Creutzfeldt-Jakob disease; TRALI = transfusion-related acute lung injury.

tion assessment of the available technologies for provision of pathogen-inactivated plasma in 1992, there being no usable technologies suitable for red cells or platelets at that time. Because the preference was for an unpooled product (so any residual infectivity was not spread between multiple doses), the choice at that time lay between quarantine plasma (ie, held in frozen storage until the donor next returns to donate and is found to have negative results for mandatory microbiologic tests on both occasions) and the MB product. (The pooled SD plasma was not licensed in the UK until autumn 1998.) Usage of plasma in Scotland has been between 25,000 and 30,000 units per year for a population of 5 million. In addition, half as much again (10,000-15,000 units) is used to prepare cryoprecipitate. For the UK as a whole, usage is about 10 times this. In developing options, it was agreed that Scotland and Northern Ireland would work together operationally (total blood donations were about 380,000 per year as compared to around 3 million for the UK as a whole), although there has been good collaboration between the four home countries in the development and validation phases.

As a precautionary measure, beginning November 1994, all plasma products were prepared from repeat donors. In 1997 the Microbiology Safety of Blood and Tissues Advisory Committee recommended a move toward virally safer plasma in the UK, though funding was not provided at that time. In response, the SNBTS undertook a validation of the Baxter PathInact system.[7] This was performed on fresh plasma, although it was later realized that the use of frozen plasma as starting material made logistics much simpler and was essential when the move to imported plasma occurred. Following this, and when funding was provided (blood transfusion was centrally funded at that time and remains so in Scotland), MB plasma was made available for children in Scotland beginning June 1998.

In early 2000 the SNBTS undertook a validation of the newly available MacoPharma system,[8] because Baxter was withdrawing from the market, and the MacoPharma system was introduced in Glasgow and Edinburgh centers beginning late summer 2000. Soon thereafter a range of methylene-blue filters became available, and these were assessed in a UK-wide study that also examined the impact of using fresh vs frozen plasma.[9] Intermediate freezing of such plasma resulted in a somewhat greater loss of coagulation activity than when fresh plasma was treated, but the MB removal filters had minimal impact on the product potency. The main effects were a loss of between 20% and 30% of Factor VIII and fibrinogen, and to address this, specifications for MB plasma differed from those for standard FFP (see section on product specification below). Beginning July 2002 the product was supplied for children in Wales and England. This was accompanied by advice to prescribing clinicians on the product and the reasons it was being made available for children in the UK.[5,6,10,11]

Precautionary Measures Addressing vCJD Concerns

In 2002 and 2003, studies in small animals demonstrated that vCJD and familial CJD could result in infectivity in the plasma component of blood.[12] Subsequently, funding was made available to import plasma for children born since December 31, 1995 (ie, those deemed not to have been exposed to infected beef) to reduce the risk of transmission of vCJD. Procuring plasma from outside the UK for this purpose proved challenging but was achieved from US donors, and supply of the product was phased in between 2003 and June 2004. Because of concerns about the differences in the prevalence of endemic viruses between exporting and importing countries, the frozen plasma was subjected to MB treatment and MB removal in the UK. (This provided helpful assurance when West Nile virus transmission became a concern in the United States.) In July 2005 the supply of this plasma was extended to all children up to the age of 16.

The UK Standing Advisory Committee on the Safety of Blood, Tissues, and Organs (SaBTO) recommended in July 2009 that all plasma used clinically in the UK should be imported from a region with low risk of vCJD.[1] This recommendation is under consideration at present. Although other approaches to pathogen inactivation of plasma are now described, including riboflavin photo-inactivation[13] and treatment with ultraviolet light,[14] only one product has so far been described that includes a specific step to remove prion infectivity.[15]

Approaches Taken for Cryoprecipitate

Many European countries no longer supply cryoprecipitate, but it is still used fairly extensively in the UK (and some Scandinavian countries), where, unlike many European countries, there is no licensed fibrinogen concentrate. Despite the loss of Factor VIII and fibrinogen in MB plasma, the SNBTS demonstrated it was possible to prepare cryoprecipitate from it,[7,16] although, again, a revised specification has been introduced recently (Table 10-2). The SNBTS also showed in 2004 that by conditioning the plasma during frozen storage, it was possible to enhance the fibrinogen, but not the Factor VIII, content of the product.[18]

Thrombotic Thrombocytopenic Patients and Adult Plasma Recipients

Observational studies have reported for some time that MB plasma is possibly less effective than other types of plasma for the treatment of TTP by plasma exchange.[10] Recently a multicenter cohort study comparing MB and quarantine plasma has confirmed that use of MB plasma is associated with a greater volume of plasma use, less-

Table 10-2. UK Specifications for Standard and MB Plasma and Cryoprecipitate*

Product	Factor VIII Content	Fibrinogen Content
Standard FFP	>0.7 IU/mL	Not specified
Standard cryoprecipitate	>70 IU per single donation component	>140 mg per single donation component
MB FFP	>0.5 IU/mL	Not specified
MB cryoprecipitate	>50 IU per single donation component	>140 mg per single donation component

*For these specifications, 75% of units should comply.[17]
MB = methylene-blue (treated); FFP = fresh frozen plasma.

frequent remission of TTP by day 8, and a higher frequency of recrudescence.[19] The mechanism of TTP is thought to involve deficiency of, or presence of antibody to, an enzyme that cleaves von Willebrand factor multimers (ADAMTS-13), with therapeutic plasma exchange allowing normalization of enzyme levels. The observation of reduced effectiveness of MB plasma remains curious inasmuch as studies have reported that MB plasma contains normal levels of ADAMTS-13.[20]

Because of this disadvantage of MB plasma, SD plasma sourced from outside the UK (and screened by nucleic acid tests for two nonenveloped viruses for which SD treatment is not effective—parvovirus B19 and hepatitis A virus) has been recommended by the Departments of Health for UK patients undergoing large-volume plasma exchange therapy.[21] In practice this mainly involves individuals with TTP. It has also been reported that pooled SD plasma is not associated with the development of transfusion-related acute lung injury (TRALI),[5] whereas apheresis plasma, particularly that from multiparous female donors, has been associated with TRALI.

Product Demand in Scotland and Northern Ireland

As shown in Fig 10-1, overall demand for MB plasma and cryoprecipitate in Scotland and Northern Ireland has been fairly steady at about 2000 units per year. Approximately half of this has been in the form of cryoprecipitate used chiefly for treatment of acquired fibrinogen deficiency. These figures represent about 3% or 4% of the overall demand in the UK for plasma and cryoprecipitate in all age groups of patients.

Product Specification, Validation, and Licensing

For normal FFP and cryoprecipitate in the UK, specifications require that 75% of the units of plasma should contain at least 0.7 IU/mL of Factor VIII, and 75% of cryoprecipitate units should contain at least 70 IU of Factor VIII and 140 mg of fibrinogen.[17] For the MB products this specification was reduced to 0.5 IU/mL and 50 IU of Factor VIII for plasma and cryoprecipitate, respectively, but with no change in

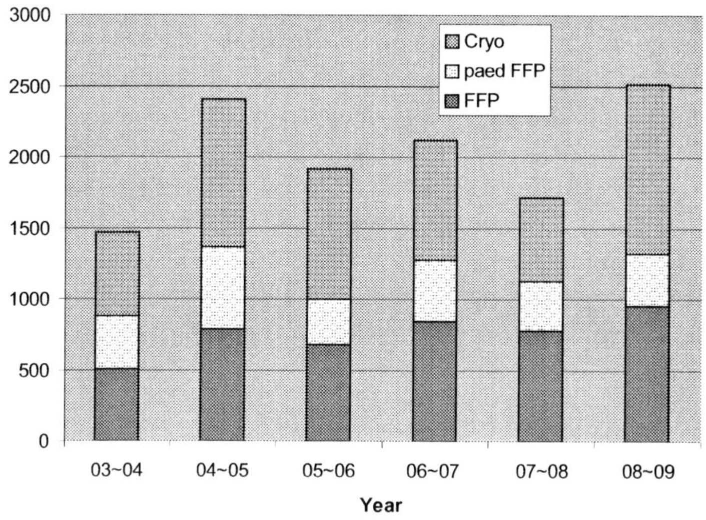

Figure 10-1. Number of full-size MB plasma units (~280 mL), pediatric-dose MB plasma units (~4 × 70 mL), and cryoprecipitate units (derived from MB plasma) issued by year for Scotland and Northern Ireland from 2003 to 2009. Overall UK figures are approximately 10-fold higher. Cryo = cryoprecipitate; paed = pediatric; FFP = fresh frozen plasma.

the fibrinogen content requirement.[21] Quality control data for production in Scotland over the period shown in Fig 10-1 demonstrate that imported frozen plasma from the United States contained, on average, 0.98 IU/mL of Factor VIII. This was reduced to 0.72 IU/mL by MB treatment and removal—ie, a 27% loss as compared to a loss of 10% to 20% when unfrozen plasma is treated. For cryoprecipitate over the same period, the average content was 82 IU Factor VIII and 229 mg fibrinogen. Other than occasional studies taken on individual viruses, the author is not aware of any independent, published, formal validation studies of virus inactivation for MB plasma. Hence one must rely on the manufacturer's data or that of its partners[2-4] to ensure viral safety.[5,10]

In Europe, single-donation blood components and small pools of these are covered by medical devices legislation. The process of CE marking (Conformité Européenne, a European license to market within the European Union) under this legislation largely assesses the manufacturer's ability to consistently provide a process and device that yields a product (rather than the product per se) that meets a specification set by the manufacturer. This may include an element of clinical evidence. Some European countries require that individual components also be licensed at a national level (eg, France: MB plasma licensed in August 2005) or a regional level (eg. Germany: MB plasma licensed in 2007). The MacoPharma Macotronic system for preparation of apheresis MB plasma was granted the CE mark in 2001 *as a medical device.* Current legislation in the UK does not require single-donation blood components to have a product license.

References

1. Advisory Committee on the Safety of Blood, Tissues and Organs (SaBTO). Summary of the Seventh Meeting, 14/15 July 2009. London: SaBTO, 2009. [Available at: http://www.dh.gov.uk/prod_consum_dh/groups/dh_digitalassets/@dh/@ab/documents/digitalasset/dh_103852.pdf, via http://www.dh.gov.uk/ab/SaBTO/index.htm (accessed May 12, 2010).]
2. Lambrecht B, Mohr H, Knüver-Hopf J, Schmitt H. Photoinactivation of viruses in human fresh plasma by phenothiazine dyes in combination with visible light. Vox Sang 1991;60:207-13.
3. Mohr H, Lambrecht B, Knuever-Hopf J. Virus inactivated single-donor fresh plasma preparations. Infusionsther Transfusionsmed 1992;19:79-83.
4. Mohr H, Bachmann B, Klein-Struckmeier A, Lambrecht B. Virus inactivation of blood products by phenothiazine dyes and light. Photochem Photobiol 1997;65:441-5.
5. Prowse C. Pathogen inactivated plasma. Transfus Med Rev 2009;23:124-33.
6. Prowse CV. Pathogen inactivation of blood components. Transfus Altern Transfus Med 2008;10:139-46.
7. Hornsey VS, Kraildsiri P, MacDonald S, et al. Coagulation factor content of cryoprecipitate prepared from methylene blue plus light virus-inactivated plasma. Br J Haematol 2000;109:665-70.
8. Hornsey VS, Drummond O, Young D, et al. A potentially improved approach to methylene–blue virus inactivation of plasma: The Maco Pharma Macotronic system. Transfus Med 2001;11:31-6.
9. Garwood M, Cardigan R, Drummond O, et al. The effect of methylene blue photoinactivation and methylene blue removal on the quality of fresh frozen plasma. Transfusion 2003;43:1238-47.
10. Williamson LM, Cardigan R, Prowse CV. Methylene blue treated fresh frozen plasma: What is its contribution to blood safety? Transfusion 2003;43:1322-9.

11. Cardigan R, Prowse C, Williamson LM. Processing of components: Leucodepletion and pathogen reduction. In: Barbara JAJ, Contreras MC, Regan FAM, eds. Transfusion microbiology. Cambridge, UK: Cambridge University Press, 2008:239-58.
12. Cervenakova L, Yakovleva O, McKenzie C, et al. Similar levels of infectivity in the blood of mice infected with human-derived vCJD and GSS strains of transmissible spongiform encephalopathy. Transfusion 2003;43:1687-94.
13. Hornsey VS, Drummond O, Morrison A, et al. Pathogen reduction of fresh plasma using riboflavin and UV light: Effects on plasma coagulation proteins. Transfusion 2009;49:2167-72.
14. Mohr H, Gravemann U, Müller TH. Inactivation of pathogens in single units of therapeutic fresh plasma by irradiation with ultraviolet light. Transfusion 2009;49:2144-51.
15. Heger A, Svae TE, Neisser-Svae A, et al. Biochemical quality of the pharmaceutically licensed plasma Octaplas LG after implementation of a novel prion protein (PrPsc) removal technology and reduction of the solvent/detergent (S/D) process time. Vox Sang 2009;97:219-25.
16. Hornsey V, Young D, Prowse C. Cryoprecipitate prepared from methylene-blue treated fresh plasma. Transfusion 2001;41:151-2.
17. Specifications for blood components: Table 8.19 (Fresh frozen plasma, neonatal use, methylene blue treated and removed, leucocyte depleted) and Table 8.20 [(Change Notification No. 3—2009) Cryoprecipitate, methylene blue treated and removed, leucocyte depleted]. In: Guidelines for the Blood Transfusion Services in the UK. 7th ed. London: UK Blood Transfusion Services, 2005. [Available at: http://www.transfusionguidelines.org.uk/index.aspx?Publication=RB and http://www.transfusionguidelines.org.uk/index.aspx?Publication=RB&Section=25&pageid=606#tab8.20 (accessed May 12, 2010).
18. Hornsey VS, Young DA, Docherty A, et al. Cryoprecipitate prepared from plasma treated with methylene blue plus light: Increasing the fibrinogen concentration. Transfus Med 2004;14:369-74.
19. del Río-Garma J, Alvarez-Larrán A, Martínez C, et al. Methylene blue photoinactivated plasma versus quarantine fresh frozen plasma in thrombotic thrombocytopenic purpura: A multicentric, prospective cohort study. Br J Haematol 2008;143:39-45.
20. del Río-Garma J, Pereira A, Arroyo JL, et al for the Spanish Apheresis Group (Grupo Español de Aféresis GEA). ADAMTS-13 activity and von Willebrand factor levels in methylene-blue photo-inactivated plasma processed by either the Springe method or an "in house" system. Vox Sang 2008;95:101-5.
21. Feeley D. Availability of imported fresh frozen plasma in Scotland. NHS HDL(2006)52. (August 30, 2006) Edinburgh, UK: Scottish Executive, Health Department, 2006. [Available at http://www.sehd.scot.nhs.uk/mels/HDL2006_52.pdf; the equivalent English direction is available at http://www.dh.gov.uk/en/Publicationsandstatistics/Lettersandcirculars/Dearcolleagueletters/DH_4127673 (accessed May 12, 2010).]

In: AuBuchon JP, Prowse CV, eds.
Pathogen Inactivation: The Penultimate Paradigm Shift
Bethesda, MD: AABB Press, 2010

11

Spain: Methylene-Blue Plasma

MIGUEL LOZANO, MD, PHD, AND
JOAN CID, MD, PHD

IN SPAIN IN JUNE 1998, AN ORDER OF THE MINISTRY of Health and Consumers enforced measures to increase the safety of fresh frozen plasma (FFP) devoted to transfusion. The measures were to be implemented by October 11, 1998.[1] The three proposed approaches established in the order as acceptable were the transfusion of 1) FFP units from the same donations as any Red Blood Cell (RBC) units or platelet concentrates that had already been transfused to the

---

Miguel Lozano, MD, PhD, Acting Chief, Hemotherapy Section, and Joan Cid, MD, PhD, Hematologist, Department of Hemotherapy and Hemostasis, Hospital Clínic, Institut d'Investigacions Biomèdiques August Pi i Sunyé, Barcelona, Spain

M. Lozano has disclosed financial relationships with Cerus and CaridianBCT. J. Cid has disclosed no conflicts of interest.

patient (shared FFP), 2) quarantine FFP (in which case the donor had been retested before transfusion of the plasma), or 3) inactivated FFP. The order listed two methods for inactivating FFP: methylene blue (MB) and light treatment and solvent/detergent (SD) treatment; however, because at that time only MB was approved in Spain, this was the method of inactivation used by those who began applying a pathogen-inactivation method to FFP.

The approaches finally chosen and implemented by the 17 different autonomous regions in Spain varied. Catalonia had already decided in July 1997 to implement MB inactivation of all FFP for transfusion. (At that time, Catalonia had about 6,000,000 inhabitants and collected about 200,000 whole blood donations per year.) Some (Aragón, Asturias, Catalonia, Extremadura, Galicia, and La Rioja) completely implemented FFP pathogen-inactivated with MB, while others (Baleares, Cantabria, Madrid, and Comunidad Valenciana) combined MB pathogen inactivation and quarantine, and still others set up a system for FFP for transfusion based exclusively on quarantine (Andalucía, Murcia, Navarra, and País Vasco). As a whole, of the 57,000 liters of FFP used for transfusion in Spain in 2005, about 63% were pathogen-inactivated with MB and 37% were transfused using a quarantine protocol.[2]

Methylene-Blue Treatment Methods

There are two systems available in Spain for treating FFP for transfusion with MB. The most frequently used approach is to send the FFP units to an external facility where individual bags undergo MB treatment according to the Springe method (Biomat Grífols, Parets del Vallés, Spain). After treatment, the units are returned to the blood center that sent them, for distribution. The alternative is to apply the treatment "in house" with the kits available from two manufacturers (Fenwal or MacoPharma). The main difference between the two systems lies in the fact that because the dye has a low capacity for entering the lymphocytes, these are destroyed by the freeze-thaw step in the Springe method, and thus the intracellular pathogens are exposed to the effect of MB. By contrast, the in-house methods remove the lymphocytes by filtration, thus reducing the amount of pathogens potentially present in the plasma after later freezing and thawing. The use of filters after MB treatment that are capable of removing the residual MB to almost undetectable levels and causing minor reductions in coagulation factor levels[3,4] is not currently a common practice in Spain.

Both MB methods are easily incorporated into the working schedule of blood transfusion centers, and given the long shelf-life of FFP, the inactivation process does not affect stock management of the product. In Spain, the price of an FFP unit (with a volume of around 220 mL) treated with MB for a transfusion service varies among the different autonomous regions using these pathogen-inactivation methods—between 48 and 55.4 euros.

Dosing-Related Concerns

Following the results of several in-vitro studies showing a decrease in coagulation factor activity after MB treatment,[5,6] there was some concern about a potential increase in the number of FFP units that might need to be transfused to achieve an equivalent clinical effect. For example, Atance et al reported in 2001 that the introduction of MB-treated FFP was associated with a 56% increase in the aggregated demand for plasma, and the transfusion of non-virus-inactivated cryoprecipitate increased twofold the first year and threefold the second year. The growth in the use of FFP was observed in all the diagnostic categories examined.[7]

Interestingly, this increase in the consumption of plasma seen in one institution was not observed when all Catalonia was taken into account. Fig 11-1 shows the evolution in FFP consumption expressed as total units transfused and the ratio between FFP units transfused per 100 RBC units in Catalonia from 1991 to 2004. Because of the perceived overtransfusion of FFP in Spain (ratios of about 50 FFP units/100 RBC units reported[2]), the Ministry of Health held a consensus conference where representatives of different medical specialty societies gathered to create guidelines for the optimal usage of FFP. The results of this consensus conference were published in 1993 in several Spanish journals in order to ensure their maximum dissemination.[8] As a consequence, a tendency toward decreased usage observed in early 1990s continued in Catalonia, reaching rates of about 16 FFP units/100 RBC units. This value did not change significantly after the introduction of MB.[9] A similar scenario was observed when the figures for FFP usage from all of

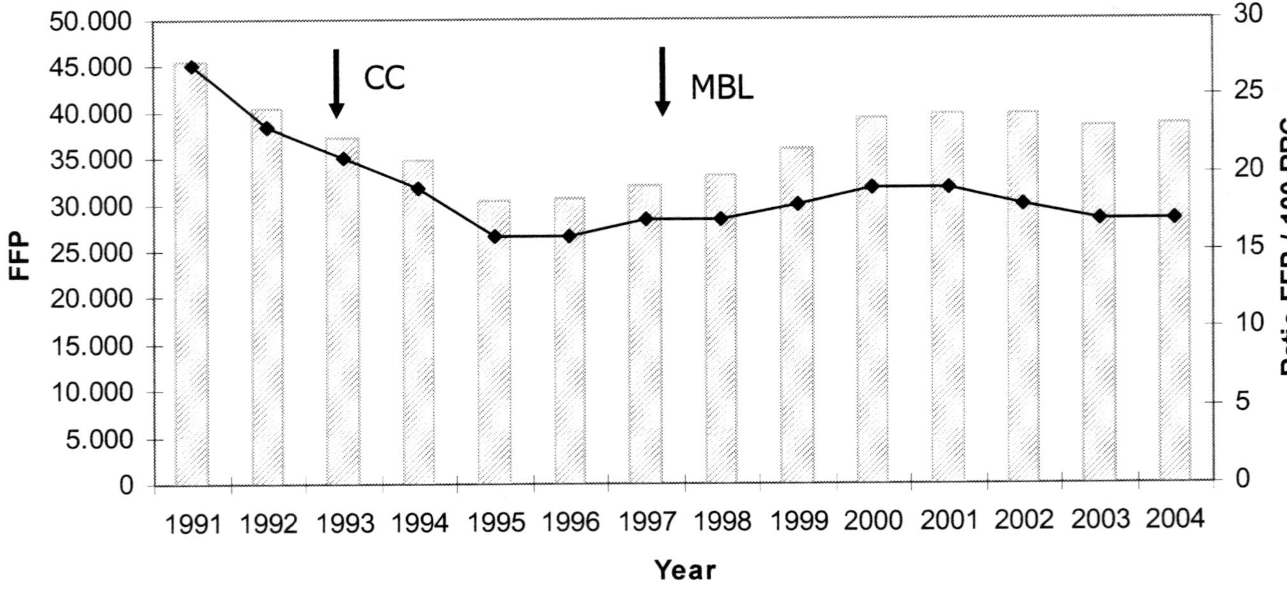

Figure 11-1. Evolution of fresh frozen plasma (FFP) consumption in Catalonia. Bars represent the number of units (left y axis) transfused every year, and the line, the ratio of FFP units transfused per 100 Red Blood Cell (RBC) units (right y axis). In 1993 a consensus conference (CC) about the clinical indications of FFP was published, and in late 1997 methylene blue/light (MBL) treatment was introduced in Catalonia for all FFP units for transfusion.

Spain were considered.[2] (However, in the case of the entire country, only about 63% of the FFP transfused had been treated with MB, in contrast to Catalonia, where 100% of FFP was being treated with MB.)

Concerns Related to Treatment of Thrombotic Thrombocytopenic Purpura

Another issue related to MB-treated FFP in Spain that has received close attention is its use as a replacement solution in plasma exchanges for treating thrombotic thrombocytopenic purpura (TTP). In 2001, de la Rubia et al published their experience treating TTP with plasma exchanges using MB-treated FFP as a replacement solution. They reported the results of the treatment of 13 patients before introducing MB-treated FFP, and seven patients after its introduction; the groups were similar in their clinical characteristics.[10] The complete remission rate was higher in the group receiving standard FFP in comparison to MB FFP (69% vs 57%; p value not reported). The mean number of procedures was higher in MB FFP (21 ±7 vs 11 ±3; p = 0.01), and the mean duration of hospitalization was also longer (37 ±12 days vs 22 ±11 days; p = 0.01). Mortality was similar in the two groups. Álvarez-Larrán et al performed a retrospective study of patients treated between 1990 and 2003 in eight Spanish hospitals. They analyzed the patients in terms of episodes of TTP, 29 occurring with standard FFP before introducing MB FFP as a replacement solution for plasma exchanges, and 27 occurring afterward.[11] The authors used a multivariate logistic regression analysis and found that the patients treated with MB FFP had an increased risk of dying from progressive TTP [adjusted odds ratio (OR) = 31; 95% confidence interval (CI): 1.2 to >100], a greater number of recurrences while on plasma exchange therapy (OR = 4·6; 95% CI: 1.2-17), and a lower probability of attaining a sustained remission within 9 days of starting plasma exchange (OR = 5.2; 95% CI:1.3-20).

In 2008, results were published for a Spanish multicenter prospective cohort study comparing MB FFP and quarantine FFP in the treatment of TTP. It included 102 episodes of idiopathic TTP; MB FFP was used in 63, and quarantine FFP in 39. Patients treated with MB FFP required more plasma exchanges (median = 11 vs 5; p = 0.002) and a larger volume of plasma (median = 485 mL/kg vs 216 mL/kg; p = 0.007) to achieve a remission and presented more recrudescences while on plasma exchange therapy than those receiving quarantine FFP (29 of 63 vs 8 of 39; p = 0.02).[12] The same groups tried to discover the reason for the different patterns of response observed between use of MB FFP and use of quarantine FFP as a replacement fluid for plasma exchanges, and they looked at the levels of ADAMTS-13 (a disintegrin and metalloproteinase with thrombospondin motifs) in both types of FFP. They found that the activity of ADAMTS-13 was unmodified by MB treatment, using either the Springe method or the in-house method developed by Maco-Pharma,[13] as reported in the past by others measuring activity or antigenicity.[14,15]

Although all the studies performed in Spain have been observational, their repeated findings seem to suggest that MB FFP is less effective than nontreated FFP in the treatment of TTP. Nevertheless, because different types of biases cannot completely be ruled out in cohort studies (selection, observational, etc), probably only a randomized controlled trial of sufficient power would clarify the utility of MB FFP in the treatment of TTP.

Adverse Events

Hemovigilance data suggest that the side effects associated with the use of MB FFP are similar to those seen with standard FFP. In the 2007 Spanish hemovigilance report, 313 allergic reactions were reported, with FFP involved in 34% of them; a similar percentage (31%) was published in the report for 2006.[16] In Catalonia, where 100% of transfused FFP is treated with MB, the percentage was similar (32%). Of the 12 cases of transfusion-related acute lung injury reported in Catalonia, MB FFP had been transfused in four (alone in one and with RBCs in three). No other severe reactions were reported.[17]

References

1. Ministerio de Sanidad y Consumo. Orden de 2 de junio de 1998 por la que se establecen principios de actuación dirigidos a la seguridad del plasma para uso transfusional. Boletín Oficial del Estado 1998:19293-4.

2. Algora M, Barbolla L. Uses of plasma in Spain. Transfus Clin Biol 2007;14: 564-7.
3. AuBuchon JP, Pickard C, Herschel L, et al. Removal of methylene blue from plasma via an adsorbent filter. Vox Sang 1998;74:1-6.
4. Riggert J, Humpe A, Legler TJ, et al. Filtration of methylene blue-photooxidized plasma: Influence on coagulation and cellular contamination. Transfusion 2001;41:82-6.
5. Zeiler T, Riess H, Wittmann G, et al. The effect of methylene blue phototreatment on plasma proteins and in vitro coagulation capability of single-donor fresh-frozen plasma. Transfusion 1994;34:685-9.
6. Aznar JA, Bonanad S, Montoro JM, et al. Influence of methylene blue photoinactivation treatment on coagulation factors from fresh frozen plasma, cryoprecipitates and cryosupernatants. Vox Sang 2000;79:156-60.
7. Atance R, Pereira A, Ramirez B. Transfusing methylene blue-photoinactivated plasma instead of FFP is associated with an increased demand for plasma and cryoprecipitate. Transfusion 2001;41:1548-52.
8. Conferencia de consenso: Indicaciones clínicas y riesgos del plasma fresco congelado. Sangre 1993;38:259-64.
9. Solheim BG, Cid J, Osselaer JC. Pathogen reduction technologies. In: Lozano M, Contreras M, Blajchman M, eds. Global perspectives in transfusion medicine. Bethesda, MD: AABB Press, 2006:103-48.
10. de la Rubia J, Arriaga F, Linares D, et al. Role of methylene blue-treated or fresh-frozen plasma in the response to plasma exchange in patients with thrombotic thrombocytopenic purpura. Br J Haematol 2001;114:721-3.
11. Alvarez-Larran A, Del Rio J, Ramirez C, et al. Methylene blue-photoinactivated plasma vs fresh-frozen plasma as replacement fluid for plasma exchange in thrombotic thrombocytopenic purpura. Vox Sang 2004;86:246-51.
12. del Río Garma J, Alvarez-Larran A, Martinez C, et al. Methylene blue-photoinactivated plasma versus quarantine fresh frozen plasma in thrombotic thrombocytopenic purpura: A multicentric, prospective cohort study. Br J Haematol 2008;143:39-45.
13. del Río Garma J, Pereira A, Arroyo JL, et al. ADAMTS-13 activity and von Willebrand factor levels in methylene-blue photo-inactivated plasma processed by either the Springe method or an 'in house' system. Vox Sang 2008; 95:101-5.
14. Cardigan R, Allford S, Williamson L. Levels of von Willebrand factor-cleaving protease are normal in methylene blue-treated fresh-frozen plasma. Br J Haematol 2002;117:253-4.
15. Cid J, Ramiro L, Martinez N, et al. Quantitative and qualitative analysis of proteins in fresh frozen plasma obtained from whole blood donations and prepared with two photochemical treatments. Transfus Apher Sci 2008;39: 115 21.
16. Informe hemovigilancia 2007. Madrid: Ministerio de Sanidad y Política Social, Area de hemoterapia, 2009. [Available at http://www.msps.es/profesionales/saludPublica/medicinaTransfusional/publicaciones/publicaciones.htm (accessed May 12, 2010).]

17. L'Hemovigilància a Catalunya. Informe 2007. Barcelona: Department de Salut, Generalitat de Catalunya, 2009. [Available at http://www.bancsang.net/ca/receptors/hemovigilancia.html (accessed May 12, 2010).]

In: AuBuchon JP, Prowse CV, eds.
Pathogen Inactivation: The Penultimate Paradigm Shift
Bethesda, MD: AABB Press, 2010

12

France: Intercept Platelets and Plasma

JEAN-PIERRE CAZENAVE, MD, PHD; HERVÉ ISOLA; CHANTAL WALLER, MD; AND DANIEL KIENTZ, MD

THE FRENCH BLOOD TRANSFUSION SERVICE (ETABlissement Français du Sang, EFS) is a national public service under the control of the Ministry of Health and the sole operator of blood collection establishments in France. It is composed of headquarters and 17 regional blood centers (14 in metropolitan France and 3 overseas). EFS has responsibility for providing a safe and adequate blood supply and for preparing labile blood products (LBPs).

Jean-Pierre Cazenave, MD, PhD, Director; Hervé Isola, Biotechnology Engineer and Chief, Component Laboratory; Chantal Waller, MD, Chief, Hemovigilance; and Daniel Kientz, MD, Chief, Distribution of Blood Components, Etablissement Français du Sang Alsace, Strasbourg, France

J. P. Cazenave has disclosed a financial relationship with Cerus. H. Isola, C. Waller, and D. Kientz have disclosed no conflicts of interest.

Over the last decade, EFS Alsace, one of the regional centers, has gained extensive experience with pathogen inactivation (PI) of platelet concentrates (PCs) and plasma. The president of EFS decided that this center should play the role of pilot center for the implementation of PI in France in testing new inactivation techniques, in providing resources to implement PI in other regional EFS centers, and in serving as a model region converted to the inactivation of PCs and plasma for 100% of production.

The reasons that led EFS Alsace to become interested in studying methods of PI in LBPs and their effective implementation include the following goals:

- To achieve greater transfusion safety through a proactive rather than reactive approach.
- To reduce bacterial contamination of PCs.
- To reduce the transmission of tested and undetected viruses as a result of the serologic window, the low number of copies, and mutations.
- To inactivate new untested or emerging pathogens [eg, cytomegalovirus (CMV), West Nile virus, chikungunya virus, dengue virus, H1N1 and H5N1 influenza, *Trypanosoma cruzi* (agent of Chagas disease), malaria, *Leishmania*, Q fever].
- To reduce morbidity and mortality.
- To satisfy the basic therapeutic and pharmaceutical principle that any product administered to patients intravenously should be sterile and apyrogenic or have undergone pathogen-inactivating or attenuating treatments.

PI using amotosalen hydrochloride and ultraviolet A (UVA) irradiation (Intercept Blood System, Cerus Corp, Concord, CA) was approved in France by the regulatory authority, Agence Française de Sécurité Sanitaire des Produits de Santé (AFSSAPS), in 2003 for PCs both from apheresis and from pooled, whole-blood, leukocyte-reduced, standard buffy-coat platelets inactivated by amotosalen. Intercept plasma collected by apheresis and leukocyte reduced was approved in 2007.

Intercept Implementation in France

The LBPs treated by Intercept (apheresis PCs, standard buffy-coat PCs, and plasma) and approved by the AFSSAPS are deemed to be not clinically different from PCs or FFP not treated by PI. Thus their clinical indications are for patients requiring PCs or fresh frozen plasma (FFP) according to French good clinical practices.

At the present time, universal (100%) transfusion of Intercept PCs is performed only in four regional EFS centers, and Intercept plasma, in six regional EFS centers and in the army transfusion center. Since 2006, Intercept has been implemented in Alsace, first as a pilot validation center for PCs and plasma and then as a region totally converted to PI. Alsace helped implement PI for PCs (Intercept apheresis PCs) during the chikungunya epidemic at EFS-Ile de la Réunion in 2006[1] and in 2007 at EFS-Martinique and EFS-Guadeloupe-Guyane during the dengue epidemic and because of high prevalence of *T. cruzi*. This strategy was applied to test the feasibility of universal use of PI under routine operating conditions as recommended by the Toronto consensus conference.[2]

Operational Experience in Preparing Intercept Platelets and Plasma

The Intercept Blood System, combining amotosalen and UVA, enables PI of PCs and therapeutic plasma with the use of a single illumination system.[3] Intercept inactivates a broad spectrum of pathogenic agents,[4] such as enveloped and nonenveloped viruses, gram-negative and gram-positive bacteria (both aerobic and anaerobic), parasites, and spirochetes, bringing about a reduction of infectivity on the order of 5 to 6 $\log_{10}$. This technique likewise inactivates with the same efficacy the intracellular viruses human immunodeficiency virus, human T-cell lymphotropic virus, CMV, and hepatitis B virus when administered in vivo to the chimpanzee. The inactivation of residual T lymphocytes ($\geq 5 \log_{10}$) makes it possible to eliminate gamma irradiation for PCs and plasma treated by Intercept.

The implementation of Intercept at EFS Alsace was preceded by an outfitting of the LBP preparation premises in January 2006. The production flow was maintained, and the inactivation room for PCs and plasma includes bench top space for four illuminators and, on the other side, two platelet agitators at 22 ±2 C (one for buffy coats and one for apheresis units). From December 2005 to January 2006, all 10 preparation technicians were trained in PI for PCs and plasma using Intercept. In parallel, from January to April 2006 and subsequently, information was disseminated in Alsace to prescribing doctors, the directors of hospitals, and the regional medical inspectors of the health ministry via conferences and written documents.

The replacement of PCs prepared in plasma with PCs prepared in additive solution [T-Sol, (Baxter International, Deerfield, IL)] and then the introduction of PI was phased in over a period of nearly 2 years. The production of noninactivated PCs in 100% plasma had totally stopped by September 2005, and noninactivated PCs in T-Sol continued until August 2006. Pathogen-inactivated products were phased in over this period: all buffy-coat-sourced PCs throughout Alsace (a region of about 2,000,000 inhabitants with three major public hospitals) were inactivated by May 9, 2006, and all apheresis units, by July 20, 2006.

The routine production (100%) of PI plasma from apheresis plasma, treated and frozen within 8 hours of collection, began on July 9, 2007. When production reached 2000 units of 200-mL each, the production of quarantine FFP was halted. Since September 1, 2007, only PI apheresis plasma has been distributed in Alsace.

The consequences of the introduction of Intercept have been modest for the organization of the preparation laboratory, resulting in one additional technician for the production of LBPs (an increase from 9 to 10 technicians at 7.5 hours per day). Whole blood collection usually takes place from 3:00 pm to 9:00 pm (day 0). LBPs are prepared the next day (day 1) after the blood has been kept at 22 ±2 C overnight and tested. They are available for transfusion according to the same schedule used where only noninactivated PCs or plasma were produced—that is, on day 1 for plasma and apheresis platelets and on day 2 for red cells. For organizational reasons (not having a second work cycle at night), the PI buffy-coat platelets are available on day 2. This change in the production of PCs has not resulted in a modification in the availability of the PCs for hospitals.

The work of the technicians has been eased greatly by the halting of the CMV serology testing and gamma irradiation for Intercept PCs and plasma. Halting the quarantine approach for FFP, and replacement with PI, has improved the immediate availability and storage of the plasma (6000 units of 200-mL each without running out of stock), freeing up two secretaries for call-back of donors and freeing up space in the –30 C cold room.

Production and Characteristics of Intercept-Treated Components

Platelet Concentrates

From 2003 to 2006, the production of noninactivated platelets underwent modifications to improve the PCs, by standardizing their preparation, and to be prepared to implement PI. The course of PC preparation during these years had three phases. First, PCs were prepared in 100% plasma. Next, an additive solution (T-Sol) was introduced, manually for the buffy-coat platelets or automatically for the apheresis platelets [Haemonetics MCS+ (Braintree, MA)], so as to reduce the secondary effects associated with the plasma and to use this plasma for fractionation. Finally, the Intersol additive solution (Fenwal, Lake Zurich, IL) was used to enable PI by the Intercept system.

Characteristics of the production and distribution of PCs inactivated by Intercept are summarized below and represent a 3-year experience (2006-2009) of 100% production and clinical use of inactivated plasma and platelet components in Alsace.

The Intercept production technique was validated according to the characteristics of apheresis and buffy-coat platelets as defined by the AFSSAPS. Before treatment, the PCs should have platelet content between 2×10^{11} and 7×10^{11} platelets. Platelets are suspended in Intersol, and the residual plasma should be between 32% and 47%. The concentration of residual red cells in the PC should not exceed 4×10^{6} red cells/mL in order to guarantee an effective illumination. A disposable medical device is connected to the PC to carry out various single operations of the Intercept process: addition of amotosalen, illumination, reduction of the residual amotosalen, and storage. The mean volume loss (from retention in the tubing) during the course of the process was 24 ±4 mL, containing 0.3 $\pm 0.07 \times 10^{11}$ platelets (7.2% of the unit contents). The final concentration of amotosalen (in routine operations) varies between 130 μM and 166 μM (required effective concentration = 120 μM to 180 μM). The illumination operation is performed under agitation and can provide an energy dose, by UVA radiation, between 3.2 and 4.3 J/cm^2. Two PCs are treated at the same time for an illumination cycle between 4 and 6 minutes. The residual amotosalen and the photoproducts are then eliminated by contact with adsorbent beads immobilized in a bag containing the PC. This operation is performed under agitation for at least 4 to 6 hours, with a maximal duration of 16 hours. The concentration of residual amotosalen should be ≤2 μM. The PC resulting from this phase is kept in a platelet storage bag (1.3 L) until the transfusion.

The set target is to prepare units containing $4 \pm 0.5 \times 10^{11}$ platelets per unit of 300 to 330 mL. More recently, the use of the TACSI centrifuge (Terumo, Tokyo, Japan) has made it possible to automate the production of buffy-coat pools and to produce a therapeutic unit with buffy coats from 5 instead of 6 units and with the same platelet content, 4×10^{11}. The platelet content of every PC is measured, and thus the exact dose administered to the patient is known. This systematic control of the buffy-coat and apheresis platelets lets one track the platelet content over the course of time, the frequency of use for each type of PC, and the distribution of the ABO groups. From 2006 to 2009, the production of Intercept PCs was 43% apheresis and 57% buffy coat platelets (of 42,560 total units). During these 3 years, the average day of delivery or distribution of Intercept PCs has been almost identical for both (Table 12-1).

Quality control testing of the Intercept PCs is performed at the preparation laboratory at the time of delivery of the product and four times a year by the AFSSAPS. Every day, the preparation laboratory tracks (for all units) the volume, the platelet concentration, and the platelet content throughout production. Residual amotosalen is measured by sampling 1% of the units produced by a validated high-performance liquid chromatography technique. The residual level of amotosalen is less (0.29 ±0.07 μM; n = 215) than the required standard of 2 μM maximum. At day 2, pH has consistently been 7.2 ±0.1 (n = 1008). The technician who delivers the Intercept PCs systematically verifies the swirling of the platelets, and only PCs demonstrating swirling (99%) are distributed. Although Intercept PCs have an allowed shelf-life of 5 days, less than 0.5% of both buffy-coat and apheresis platelet units have been outdated. Aerobic and anaerobic bacteria checks (n = 98) performed at the request of the hemovigilance officer or on outdated PCs (on day 6 or 7) have all found units to be negative through 7 days of culture.

Table 12-1. Characteristics of Intercept-Treated Platelets Prepared at EFS-Alsace*

		Buffy-Coat Platelets	
Characteristic (Amotosalen-Treated Units)	**Apheresis Platelets**	**6-Unit Pool, Manual Preparation**	**5-Unit Pool, Automated Preparation**
Total units	14,664	21,658	4163
Volume (mL)	336 ±2 (336; 20-389)	313 ±20 (311; 135-390)	303 ±16 (304; 209-382)
pH at day 2	7.2 ±0.1	7.2 ±0.1	7.2 ±0.1
Platelet content (× 10^{11}/unit)	3.9 ±0.8 (3.9; 0.2-6.0)	4.6 ±0.7 (4.6; 0.7-7.3)	4.0 ±0.7 (4.0; 1.4-6.3)
Day of issue	2.8 ±1.1 (2.8; 0.4-5.8)	3.1 ±1.0 (3.0; 1.2-5.8)	—

*Values are mean ± standard deviation (median; range). All platelet components are leukocyte reduced.

Plasma

The Intercept production technique of PI apheresis plasma was validated by the AFSSAPS, and its characteristics defined. Before treatment, the plasma volume should be between 385 and 650 mL, and residual red cells should not exceed 4×10^6/mL. A disposable medical device is connected to the plasma to carry out single operations of the process: addition of amotosalen, illumination, reduction of the residual amotosalen, freezing, and storage. The addition of 15 mL of 6 mM amotosalen HCl occurs when the plasma is transferred into the illumination bag. The concentration of amotosalen varies between 135 μM and 225 μM. The illumination operation is performed under agitation and can provide an energy dose, by UVA radiation, between 5.8 and 7.0 J/cm^2. Two plasma bags of 650 mL (maximum), collected by apheresis (Haemonetics MCS+), are treated for an illumination cycle between 6 and 8 minutes. The residual amotosalen is then eliminated by contact adsorption with adsorbent beads immobilized in a filter. This operation is accomplished (less than 30 minutes) through transfer by gravity of the illuminated plasma from the illumination bag to the three preservation bags, yielding 3 therapeutic units of ≤200 mL. The concentration of residual amotosalen should be ≤2 μM. These units should be frozen within 8 hours from the time of blood donation.

The characteristics of the Intercept plasma, in terms of hemostatic protein concentration during storage at ≤–25 C for up to 1 year, have been validated at three European transfusion centers in Germany, Norway, and France,[5] and all are in acceptable therapeutic range, with a maximal loss ≤30% for Factor VIII.

In Alsace from September 2007 to May 2009, 39,026 therapeutic units of PI apheresis plasma have been produced with a mean volume of 204 ±8 mL. The stock levels [type A (41%), B (11%), O (31%), AB (14%)] are defined so as to ensure the availability of necessary types and have been set at a total of 6000 units (12 weeks' worth of use). At EFS Alsace, in order to reduce the occurrence of transfusion-related acute lung injury (TRALI), only male plasma is used.

Quality control for this component is performed at the preparation laboratory and by the AFSSAPS. The preparation laboratory tracks (for all units) the weight of the plasma units and red cell contamination (≤4×10^6 red cells/mL) using a visual aid composed of a series of pictures of bags containing increasing concentrations of red cells to facilitate visual control. The residual level of amotosalen is ≤0.66 ±0.1 μM (n = 153). The level of Factor VIII is systematically checked by the AFSSAPS on random samples of mixtures of 6 Intercept plasma units. From 2006 to 2009, 49 pools were tested; the mean level was 0.8 ±0.1 U/mL of Factor VIII (vs the required concentration of ≥0.7 U/mL). The generation of thrombin is identical to that of plasma before inactivation.[6]

Cost

The cost of introducing Intercept to inactivate PCs and plasma units remains an important consideration for the health authorities, particularly if extension of the successful regional experience to the entire country is being considered. In France, when EFS decides to introduce a new LBP, it discusses with the Ministry of Health a reimbursement price for the LBP delivered to the hospitals and clinics. The price fixed by the Ministry of Health is published in the national official journal, and its application is mandatory. The price of a unit of plasma (200 mL) is 94.69 euros for plasma inactivated by solvent/detergent, methylene-blue, or Intercept technologies. The price of PCs is a function of the platelet content (a multiple of 0.5×10^{11} platelets) and is different for apheresis PCs, which are more expensive (about 40% more), than for pooled buffy-coat PCs. Today in France, the price of a conventional PC or of an Intercept PC is the same. If, following the EFS Alsace pilot experience, the implementation of Intercept platelets is extended to other regions, the ministry will have to reexamine the price of components.

An analysis of the net cost impact of introducing a common Intercept platform for platelets and plasma shows it has positive effects contributing to cost reduction. The cost of PCs can also be reduced by shifting from apheresis to pooled buffy-coat products in at least a 50/50 ratio. The use of Intersol solution saves plasma for fractionation. So far, France has avoided the introduction of bacterial detection, avoided the implementation CMV detection for allogeneic transplantation recipients, and replaced gamma irradiation for transfusion-associated graft-vs-host disease. Replacement of quarantine plasma with Intercept plasma had important logistic impacts, reducing the cost of plasma production and facilitating the use of plasma from male donors to prevent TRALI. In the future, PI may also contribute to further cost reductions by avoiding donor travel restrictions and avoiding introduction of new tests for emerging pathogens.

Clinical Experience with Transfusion of Intercept-Treated Components

Platelet Concentrates

To assess the impact of the use of platelet additive solutions and PI treatment, EFS Alsace conducted a retrospective review of PC use, red cell use, and acute transfusion-related reactions as reported to the hemovigilance office of the AFSSAPS during three different periods of about a year each, from January 2003 to August 2007 (Table 12-2). The study provided the opportunity to evaluate the effects of changes in platelet preparation in each period when implemented in routine use for support of a broad spectrum of patients. Each period included between 1600 and 2000 patients with no exclusions; patients had a median age of 63 years and represented a distribution across multiple case categories such as oncology/hematology, cardiac surgery, general surgery, and general medicine. These patients received between 9000 and 13,000 PCs (62% buffy-coat and 38% apheresis platelets) and between 17,000 and 23,000 Red Blood Cells (RBCs) in each period. This analysis was based on a comprehensive longitudinal database that tracked greater than 99% of PCs with respect to patient demographics and utilization by patients. In addition, the response to transfusion with respect to adverse outcomes was evaluated using an active hemovigilance program, with greater than 99% of transfusions reported in the EFS Alsace region.

During the three periods, the platelet content per component changed as the methods of production changed (Table 12-2). The usage of PCs was determined per patient on the basis of the number of PCs transfused and the total dose of platelets in PCs transfused per patient. Clinicians were prescribing transfusions of PCs according to AFSSAPS national guidelines, based on a recommended dose of 0.5 to 0.7 × 10^{11} platelets per 7 kg in adults and 0.5 × 10^{11} platelets per 5 to 7 kg in pediatric patients for support of thrombocytope-

Table 12-2. Platelet Concentrates Transfused* at EFS-Alsace

	Period 1: • 13 Months • PCs in 100% Plasma • 5.2×10^{11} Platelets†	Period 2: • 9 months • PCs in 65% T-Sol‡ • 4.4×10^{11} Platelets†	Period 3: • 11 months • Amotosalen-Treated PCs in 65% Intersol§ • 4.2×10^{11} Platelets†
Patients (n)	2050	1678	2069
Median age in years (minimum-maximum)	64 (<1-97)	63 (<1-99)	63 (<1-106)
Oncology/hematology	56%	51%	58%
Carciac surgery	7%	6%	6%
General medicine and surgery	37%	43%	36%
Platelet Concentrates			
Transfused units	10,629	9151	13,241
Mean units/patient	5.2	5.5	6.4
Median units/patient (minimum-maximum)	2.0 (1-104)	2.0 (1-114)	2.0 (1-289)

(Continued)

Table 12-2. Platelet Concentrates Transfused* at EFS-Alsace (Continued)

	Period 1: • **13 Months** • **PCs in 100% Plasma** • **5.2×10^{11} Platelets†**	**Period 2:** • **9 months** • **PCs in 65% T-Sol‡** • **4.4×10^{11} Platelets†**	**Period 3:** • **11 months** • **Amotosalen-Treated PCs in 65% Intersol§** • **4.2×10^{11} Platelets†**
Mean dose/patient (platelets × 10^{11})	27.1	24.1	26.9
Median dose/patient (platelets × 10^{11})	10.9 (0.2-543)	9.4 (0.2-503)	9.1 (0.5-1,302)
RBCs: mean units/patient	14.4	12.8	13.5
Patients (%) with at least one ATR	2.9	2	1.7
ATRs/1000 platelet units	5.3	2.7	1.4

*Ratio of buffy coat transfusions to apheresis platelets = 62/38.
†Mean platelet content of a PC unit.
‡Baxter International, Deerfield, IL.
§Fenwal, Lake Zurich, IL.
PC = platelet concentrate; RBC = Red Blood Cell; ATR = acute transfusion reaction.

nia. The total mean dose of Intercept PCs needed was 27.0×10^{11} platelets/patient, which is identical to that of conventional noninactivated PCs. Thus, the use of PCs inactivated by Intercept during period 3 resulted in no increase in platelet use compared to the two preceding periods, when conventional PCs in plasma or in additive solution were transfused (Table 12-2). Therefore, from a broad perspective, these PI platelets had hemostatic efficacy comparable to that of conventional PCs, at least in the sense that additional components were not required to be transfused. Furthermore, it should be noted that the mean number of RBCs transfused was not different between the 3 periods (Table 12-2). The ATRs were reported after each transfusion episode in accordance with the hemovigilance program of the AFSSAPS. ATRs attributed to apheresis and buffy-coat platelets of period 3 were reported as 1.7% per patient (1.4/1000 PCs), less than those of conventional PCs of period 2 (2.0% per patient) and period 1 (2.9% per patient). No cases of transfusion-related sepsis were reported in any period. Two severe reactions were reported across these three periods. In period 1, one death was caused by volume overload. In period 3, one case of nonfatal (grade 3) TRALI was attributed to the transfusion of an apheresis platelet unit prepared from a multiparous woman with HLA antibodies.

From this cohort of patients, the use of PCs and RBCs by intensively transfused patients with hematology-oncology disorders was examined. Approximately similar numbers of pediatric and adult patients were transfused during periods 1 (671 patients) and 3 (699). Although the number of PCs transfused per patient was higher during period 3 compared to period 1, the total dose of platelets per patient was not increased in period 3 ($46.1 \pm 86.1 \times 10^{11}$ platelets per patient) compared to period 1 ($45.3 \pm 62.8 \times 10^{11}$ platelets per patient; $p = 0.85$). There was no significant difference between the two groups in the mean quantity of RBCs transfused, respectively 15.2 and 13.6 RBCs per patient ($p = 0.10$). Similar results were seen when analyzing adult and pediatric recipients separately. Overall, hematology-oncology patients are generally more exposed to risk of hemorrhage and more serious thrombocytopenia and thus need a larger number of PC transfusions (median of four per patient) than the total population analyzed in the preceding section (median of two per patient). Nevertheless, the inactivated PC transfusions were just as effective with respect to hemostasis as the noninactivated, conventional PCs in 100% plasma. Likewise, the hematology-oncology patients do not need more RBCs than the general recipient population.

Plasma

Since September 2007, PI apheresis plasma has replaced quarantine FFP in Alsace, with important logistic advantages. The incidence of acute transfusion reactions (0.8 per 1000 plasma units) from 26,234 units of PI plasma was the same as that from transfusion of 35,064 units of quarantine FFP transfused during a similar period of observation. Both periods included a population of 42 patients treated with therapeutic plasma exchange requiring multiple exposures to large volumes of plasma. Of these, FFP was used in 17 cases and PI FFP in 25 cases, and the clinical results were similar. Among them, a subgroup of 16 patients with thrombotic microangiopathies, hemolytic uremic syndrome, and thrombotic thrombocytopenic purpura received FFP (5 patients) or PI FFP (11 patients). There was no difference between the two groups in the number of plasma exchanges per patient or the total volume of plasma transfused per patient, and the rate of remission was equivalent.[7]

Conclusion

PI of LBPs (platelets, plasma, and, it is hoped, RBCs in the near future) introduces a paradigm shift in transfusion safety. The clinical development of these new LPBs is similar to that of new drugs. The Intercept technology applied to plasma and platelets has undergone a rigorous (drug and device) program of preclinical (pharmacokinetics, toxicology, genotoxicity) and clinical development studies (four Phase III clinical trials for platelets and three for plasma), as detailed in other chapters. These trials were necessary to determine whether Intercept platelets[8-11] and plasma[12-14] were effective and equivalent to conventional components and whether their use could be extended to clinical practice. The predictive value of such trials is limited by the restricted selection of patient subjects, the rather small number of inclusions, the use of surrogate markers of hemostasis such as the corrected count increment, and the difficulty in measuring the clinical hemostasis efficacy primary endpoint despite its relevance.

After the evaluation of this new technology by clinical trials, it was thought important to gain supplemental information about the impact of Intercept on the organization of the blood transfusion center and on the patients under routine conditions using precisely known doses of platelets contained in each PC transfused and the total dose of platelets administered to each patient. These observational studies encompassed a large experience, indeed much larger than that of most clinical trials in transfusion medicine that have been used to implement major changes in transfusion practice, such as leukocyte reduction and adjustment of the transfusion threshold. The large clinical experience and hemovigilance safety studies derived from universal application of this PI technique have presented evidence that Intercept platelets are effective and safe when transfused to a large variety of pediatric and adult patients with acquired or hereditary defects (eg, Glanzmann thrombasthenia[15]) of platelet number and/or function. Effective hemostasis was obtained as reported in Mont Godinne, Belgium,[16] and in Strasbourg, France,[17] with a total platelet dose of Intercept PCs similar to that of noninactivated PCs. At the same time, the transfusion of RBCs was not increased, suggesting control of bleeding. Active hemovigilance surveillance reported that routine transfusions of plasma[18] and of Intercept PCs were well tolerated in a wide range of patients and that ATRs were infrequent and most were mild.[16,19]

References

1. Rasongles P, Angelini-Tibert MF, Simon P, et al. Transfusion of platelet components prepared with photochemical pathogen inactivation treatment during a chikungunya virus epidemic in Ile de La Réunion. Transfusion 2009; 49:1083-91.
2. Webert KE, Cserti CM, Hannon J, et al. Proceedings of a consensus conference: Pathogen inactivation—making decisions about new technologies. Transfus Med Rev 2008;22:1-34.
3. Intercept Blood System. One system—two components. Concord, CA: Cerus Corp, 2010. [Available at http://www.interceptbloodsystem.com/product_overview_one_system.html (accessed May 19, 2010).]
4. Naegelen C, Isola H, Dernis D, et al. Évolution des techniques de préparation des produits sanguins labiles (PSL): Inactivation des pathogènes dans les PSL. Transfus Clin Biol 2009;16:179-89.

5. Schlenke P, Hervig T, Isola H, et al. Photochemical treatment of plasma with amotosalen and UVA light: Process validation in three European blood centers. Transfusion 2008;48:697-705.
6. Cazenave JP, Netzer P, Schuhler S, et al. Retention of thrombin generation capacity of therapeutic apheresis plasma prepared with amotosalen and UVA light (Intercept) pathogen inactivation. Blood 2007;110:75B.
7. Kientz D, Wiesel ML, Lanois I, et al. Therapeutic plasma exchange (TPE) for thrombotic thrombocytopenic purpura (TTP) and hemolytic uremic syndrome (HUS) using plasma prepared with photochemical pathogen inactivation: A one year experience in routine practice in a regional blood center. Presented at the 14th Congress of the European Hematology Association, Berlin, Germany, June 4-7, 2009.
8. van Rhenen D, Gulliksson H, Cazenave JP, et al. Transfusion of pooled buffy coat platelet components prepared with photochemical pathogen inactivation treatment: The euroSPRITE trial. Blood 2003;101:2426-33.
9. McCullough J, Vesole DH, Benjamin RJ, et al. Therapeutic efficacy and safety of platelets treated with a photochemical process for pathogen inactivation: The SPRINT Trial. Blood 2004;104:1534-41.
10. Murphy S, Snyder E, Cable R, et al for the SPRINT Study Group. Platelet dose consistency and its effect on the number of platelet transfusions for support of thrombocytopenia: An analysis of the SPRINT trial of platelets photochemically treated with amotosalen HCl and ultraviolet A light. Transfusion 2006; 46:24-33.
11. Janetzko K, Cazenave JP, Kluter H, et al. Therapeutic efficacy and safety of photochemically treated aphaeresis platelets processed with an optimized integrated set. Transfusion 2005;45:1443-52.
12. De Alarcon P, Benjamin R, Dugdale M, et al. Fresh frozen plasma prepared with amotosalen HCl (S59) photochemical pathogen inactivation: Transfusion of patients with congenital coagulation factor deficiencies. Transfusion 2005;45:1362-72.
13. Mintz PD, Bass NM, Petz LD, et al. Photochemically treated fresh frozen plasma for transfusion of patients with acquired coagulopathy of liver disease. Blood 2006;107:3753-60.
14. Mintz PD, Neff A, MacKenzie M, et al. A randomized controlled Phase III trial of therapeutic plasma exchange with fresh frozen plasma (FFP) prepared with amotosalen and ultraviolet A light compared to untreated FFP in thrombotic thrombocytopenic purpura. Transfusion 2006;46:1693-704.
15. Cazenave JP, Wiesel ML, Mendel I, et al. Intensive and successful transfusion of pathogen inactivated Intercept platelet concentrates for major gynecological and obstetrical surgery in Glanzmann thrombasthenia type 1 with the Gypsy mutation. Vox Sang 2008;95(Suppl 1):306.
16. Osselaer JC, Messe N, Hervig T, et al. A prospective observational cohort safety study of 5106 platelet transfusions with components prepared with photochemical pathogen inactivation treatment. Transfusion 2008;48:1061-71.
17. Cazenave JP, Waller C, Mendel I, et al. Clinical experience with pathogen inactivation of platelet components for transfusion support. In: Scharf RE, ed. Progress and challenges in transfusion medicine, hemostasis and hemother-

apy. State of art 2008. 41st Congress of the German Society for Transfusion Medicine and Immunohematology. Baden-Baden, Germany: Karger, 2008: 248-63.

18. Osselaer JC, Cazenave JP, Lambermont M, et al. An active haemovigilance programme characterizing the safety profile of 7437 platelet transfusions prepared with amotosalen photochemical treatment. Vox Sang 2008;94:315-23.
19. Cazenave JP, Waller C, Kientz D, et al. An active hemovigilance program characterizing the safety profile of 7483 transfusions with plasma components prepared with amotosalen and UVA photochemical treatment. Transfusion 2010;50:1210-19.

In: AuBuchon JP, Prowse CV, eds.
Pathogen Inactivation: The Penultimate Paradigm Shift
Bethesda, MD: AABB Press, 2010

13

Belgium: Intercept Platelets

JEAN CLAUDE OSSELAER, MD, JD

TRANSFUSION IN BELGIUM IS GOVERNED BY A LAW (July 5, 1994) and the different royal decrees created to execute this law. The law defines the existence of blood transfusion establishments (BTEs), which are in charge of all aspects of the production of blood derivatives (components), and blood transfusion centers (BTCs), which can organize a part or the whole of this activity but are always associated with a BTE. The law defines the criteria establishments and centers must fulfill and specifies a certain number of requirements for donor selection, donor testing, and product

---

Jean Claude Osselaer, MD, JD, Medical Director, Mont-Godinne Blood Transfusion Establishment, Yvoir, Belgium

The author has disclosed no conflicts of interest.

qualification. The law also empowers the minister of health to issue or withdraw licenses for establishments and centers, to inspect facilities at any time, and to issue the legal requirements for donor selection or testing and product qualification. In special matters, the minister of health can seek the advice of the Superior Council of Health.

Currently 6 BTEs exist in Belgium: two huge regional centers run by the Belgian Red Cross, one small autonomous regional center, two hospital-based BTEs, and one BTE incorporated in the Belgian army. The medical directors of these BTEs are in charge of their policies. They can, under their own responsibility, introduce new technologies as long as they comply with the Belgian law and regulations and the blood product specifications given either by the minister of health or the National Institute of Social Insurance. No formal approval of new technologies is required unless the regulations state otherwise. An appropriate CE (Conformité Européenne) label is mandatory, however, and of course the directors of the BTEs remain responsible for the decisions they make.

The minister of health also defines the price of the different blood derivatives (components and products). Blood derivatives are completely reimbursed by the social insurance system in Belgium. The National Institute of Social Insurance is allowed to define additional requirements blood derivatives should meet in order to be reimbursed. There is also a special mechanism, contained in Article 56 of the law creating the National Institute of Social Insurance, to finance new technologies on a temporary basis to assess their feasibility and effectiveness. The only source of income for BTEs is the products they sell to the hospitals.

Status of Transfusion in Belgium Before 2003

Although bacteria detection of platelet products never was mandatory in Belgium, the BTE of the Flemish department of the Belgian Red Cross started bacteria detection in the late 1990s, followed 2 years later by the French-speaking department of the Belgian Red Cross. At that time, product sampling occurred shortly after production, and the samples were being incubated while the products were available for transfusion; in more than half of the cases, the sample turned out to be positive after the unit had already been transfused. Policies were not standardized within the Red Cross, and they varied with time: sampling occurred only on buffy-coat pools and apheresis products, policies on both the sampling time and the inoculum size varied, and the decision algorithm was not fully standardized. Nevertheless, as these two BTEs represent more than 90% of the platelet production in Belgium, bacterial detection came to be—in a certain sense and on a voluntary basis—a new standard of safety. In terms of product liability, the smaller BTEs had to choose: either follow the Red Cross and introduce bacteria detection or move to pathogen reduction in platelets.

Pathogen reduction was not really a new concept in Belgium. After 1993, the only available plasma in Belgium was solvent/detergent-treated (SD) plasma, collected from nonremunerated Belgian donors and treated under license by Octapharma. As for platelets, the Flemish department of the Belgian Red Cross and the pediatrics department of the University Hospital of Ghent (Belgium) had already conducted a Phase IV clinical trial.[1] In a population of 83 pediatric patients, of whom the vast majority had hemato-oncologic disease and received 500 amotosalen-treated buffy-coat pooled platelet concentrates, the investigators observed that transfusion of pediatric patients with Intercept (Cerus, Concord, CA) platelets provided therapeutic count increments. No unexpected transfusion reactions were attributed specifically to the use of Intercept platelets, and the Intercept system replaced the use of gamma irradiation for the inactivation of leukocytes.

Routine Use of Intercept for Pathogen Reduction in Platelets Beginning in 2003

In October 2003, the BTE of Mont-Godinne implemented the routine use of Intercept for pathogen reduction in platelets. This introduction was possible from a legal point of view because Intercept had received a Class III CE label at the end of 2002. Although not legally required, the approval of the technique by the AFSSAPS, the French regulatory body, was also a positive endorsement. In Belgium, each BTE can decide to introduce a new technique aimed at improving blood safety under the condition that it has an adequate CE label and is not specifically limited by regulatory texts on blood transfusion or on reimbursement of blood derivatives by social insurance. Because in 2003 there was a complete absence of any mention of pathogen reduction in platelets in regulations or in the nomenclature of the National Institute of Social Insurance, each BTE could freely choose to implement this method or not, possibly as an alternative for bacteria detection.

Mont-Godinne is a hospital-based BTE that supplies the Mont-Godinne University Hospital, a 400-bed teaching hospital with important departments of hematology and cardiovascular surgery. With an annual production of 3000 units of platelet concentrates, the BTE of Mont-Godinne is responsible for 5% of the national platelet production in Belgium. All platelets are produced on Amicus (Fenwal, Lake Zurich, IL) instrumentation; systematic use of additive solution for platelets had already been introduced in 1999. The BTE also runs the hospital blood bank, which facilitates the clinical feedback after transfusion.

The implementation of Intercept occurred smoothly after an in-vitro validation using split apheresis products[2] and ensuring adherence to the manufacturer's specifications for the input platelet product and the local quality requirements at issue. This was facilitated by a high degree of control of the plateletpheresis process, providing a good correlation between predicted yield and effective yield of the apheresis procedure, and by the fact that platelet additive solution was already in routine use. For the Intercept procedures, the platelet additive solution T-Sol only had to be replaced by InterSol. At that time, the use of Intercept required a platelet content between 2.5 and 6×10^{11} platelets in a volume of 255 to 325 mL. Less than 1% of the local production fell outside these parameters, of which almost half had a platelet content $<2.5 \times 10^{11}$ and would have been discarded anyhow, even without the use of the Intercept system. The vast majority of the products with a higher platelet yield could be made to fit the criteria through a volume reduction of the product.[3]

The Intercept process in itself caused a 12% loss in platelets as a result of the volume held back during the container-to-container transfers. The increase in workload was modest: an annual production of 3000 Intercept-treated concentrates was accomplished by an additional quarter-time technician.

The introduction of Intercept replaced gamma irradiation of platelets and CMV testing.[4] To date, more than 16,000 units of Intercept-treated platelets have been transfused at Mont-Godinne. This practice did not lead to any unexpected side effects in platelet recipients.

A preliminary analysis comparing the platelet transfusions during the 18 months before and after the introduction of Intercept[5] showed no increase in platelet needs after the introduction of pathogen reduction, not even in the subpopulation of chronically transfused hematology patients. Interestingly, there was a decrease in the reaction rate after platelet transfusions, which was not a plasma effect but specifically an Intercept effect because platelets had already been stored and transfused in additive solution for 18 months before Intercept implementation.

In June 2005, the BTE of Charleroi was the second transfusion center to adopt the routine use of Intercept. Charleroi is a small regional blood center, supplying five hospitals in the urban region of Charleroi, with a platelet production slightly higher than Mont-Godinne (3500 units per year). All platelets are produced by apheresis, but interestingly half of the procedures are run on TRIMA (CaridianBCT, Lakewood, CO) and half on Amicus. Despite this diversity in instrumentation, the implementation of Intercept was quite uneventful. In the same year, the routine use of Intercept was subsequently adopted by the BTE of St. John's Hospital (Bruges) and the BTE of the Belgian army.

At the end of 2005, more than 10% of the national production of platelets was treated with Intercept, whereas the remaining 90% produced by the two major BTEs of the Belgian Red Cross still underwent bacteria detection without pathogen inactivation. This situation was becoming a potential risk for liability, and the National Institute of Social Insurance took the initiative to assess the feasibility and the potential impact of this new technology.

National Assessment of Pathogen Reduction in Platelets Using Intercept Technology

The National Institute of Social Insurance law allows special funding through Article 56 for the evaluation of the impact and feasibility of new technologies. Early in 2006, a project was started to assess Intercept for pathogen reduction in platelets, both in terms of feasibility, platelet recovery (through the measurement of corrected count increments, or CCIs), and impact on transfusion needs. Four out of the six national BTEs participated in this study:

1. The BTE of the Flemish department of the Belgian Red Red Cross, through the BTC of Ghent (buffy-coat pools in pediatric patients).
2. The BTE of the French-speaking department of the Belgian Red Cross, through the BTC of Brussels-Hainaut (apheresis platelets and buffy-coat pools, adult patients).
3. The BTE of St John's Hospital (Bruges).
4. The BTE of Mont-Godinne (apheresis platelets, adult recipients).

Centers that had not previously implemented Intercept technology did so to participate in this study. The introduction of Intercept proved to be feasible even in the Red Cross centers that had no previous experience with the technique. No unexpected side effects were observed.

The comparison of CCIs, either on a contemporary or an historical basis, showed a tendency toward lower CCIs in the Intercept-treated platelet concentrates. These results were consistent with those already published for the two major Phase III clinical trials conducted with Intercept platelets. The impact of Intercept on CCIs varied, however, from center to center, and the reduction in CCI tended to be smaller for buffy-coat pools than for apheresis platelets.

Funding through Article 56 enabled Mont-Godinne to perform a more detailed analysis of 3 years' experience with Intercept.[6] Comparing the transfusion activity between the 3 years before (2000-2003) and the 3 years after (2003-2006) the implementation of Intercept platelets, no increase was observed in the platelet needs (after correction of the 12% platelet loss through production). The absence of any increase in platelet usage was confirmed in a population of 272 vs 276 hematology patients before and after implementation, respectively, totaling 8595 vs 9136 platelet transfusions in which comparable numbers of allo- and autografts had been performed. No systematic assessment of bleeding had taken place, but there was no increase in the red cell usage, even if the analysis was focused on hematology patients during the periods of platelet support. Furthermore, by checking the actual platelet counts at which these transfusions actually had been given, no difference in CCIs was observed. This observation allowed exclusion of a possible masking of an increase in transfusion needs through a lowering of transfusion thresholds. Finally, although gamma irradiation of platelets was stopped with the implementation of Intercept, no case of graft-vs-host disease was observed.

These findings were corroborated by the experience of the blood center in Strasbourg, France, which introduced Intercept for pathogen reduction in platelets in 2005. The platelet production of Strasbourg is fivefold that of Mont-Godinne, and the observations made in Strasbourg were very similar.

Based on the uniformly positive experience of the four participating BTEs, the task group for the assessment project recommended the implementation of Intercept on a routine basis across Belgium. The task group also expressed the hope that, should they become available, competing technologies be considered for reimbursement once Phase III and IV clinical trials become published. The Insurance Committee of the National Institute of Social Insurance endorsed these conclusions and recommended that the minister of health reimburse for pathogen reduction in platelet units in early 2007.

The Evolving Regulatory Environment

In 2004, the Ministry of Health changed its policy for pathogen reduction in plasma. Concern over transfusion-transmitted variant Creutzfeldt-Jakob disease led to the decision that only apheresis plasma should be used, with inactivation by a method to be approved by the Ministry of Health with the advice of the Superior Council of Health.

In 2004, the only approved technique for viral inactivation of apheresis plasma was Theraflex (Macopharma, Lille, France), using methylene blue and visible light. Some months after the decision to cease making SD-treated plasma from Belgian donors, SD plasma (Octaplas, originating from Austrian donors) was reintroduced into the Belgian market, no longer as a blood derivative but as a drug. In July 2007, the Superior Council of Health recommended that Intercept be authorized as an alternative for methylene-blue treatment for pathogen reduction in plasma units.

After having received the positive recommendation for reimbursement of pathogen reduction, the ministry of health asked for the advice of the Superior Council of Health on pathogen reduction in platelets as well. On August 6, 2008, the Superior Council of

Health concluded that the recent scientific knowledge and literature give sufficient proof that duly validated methods for pathogen reduction in platelets are effective techniques and offer the following benefits:

- Risk reduction for pathogens such as enveloped viruses, bacteria, and protozoa (but not for prions).
- Risk reduction for the transmission of emerging pathogens especially when not yet identified and therefore undetectable in the blood supply.
- Reduction of transfusion-transmitted influenza in case of influenza pandemics.

The Superior Council of Health recommended the general implementation of pathogen reduction in association with active hemovigilance. The council also stated that methods used for pathogen reduction should be appropriately validated in terms of safety and therapeutic efficacy.

Other potential benefits of the implementation of pathogen reduction in platelets include avoidance of the development of new screening tests for emerging pathogens and new donor deferral criteria, the elimination of existing tests such as bacteria detection or CMV and malaria serology, and avoidance of the need for gamma irradiation of platelets.

Based on this advice, a royal decree of June 28, 2009 required pathogen reduction in platelets through a validated method. In an accompanying ministerial decree of the same date, reimbursement for pathogen reduction in a standardized platelet concentrate was set at 108.20 euros. All BTEs have until the end of June 2010 to implement pathogen reduction.

Current Situation and Future Expectations

Shortly before the publication of the 2009 royal decree, the BTE of the French-speaking department of the Belgian Red Cross switched to Intercept for pathogen reduction in platelets. Gamma irradiation of these platelets was no longer required, but the final decision was left to the hospitals, who, after some months, completely abandoned gamma irradiation.

As of November 2009, five of the six BTEs in Belgium, representing half of the national platelet production, were treating their platelets with Intercept. One BTE, run by the Flemish department of the Belgian Red Cross, had not yet implemented the technique both because of organizational problems and because administrators wanted more scientific evidence. The implementation of pathogen reduction for platelets is expected be completed before the end of June 2010. Without pathogen reduction techniques, the possibility of a missed instance of bacterial contamination raises a liability issue, and thus their implementation is regarded as necessary.

The regulatory context for pathogen reduction in plasma is slightly different from platelets. Pathogen-reduced plasma is reimbursed (as a blood component) only when the plasma has been treated by a method on an approved list drawn up by the minister of health, with the advice of the Superior Council of Health. To date, only two authorized methods are included on this list: Theraflex and Intercept.

Belgium was the first country where pathogen reduction in platelet units was introduced on a routine basis in a transfusion center and where pathogen reduction has become mandatory on a national basis. At present, 50% of the national platelet production is pathogen reduced, and all of the national platelet production will be pathogen reduced at the latest by the middle of 2010.

To date, all platelet pathogen-reduction procedures have been performed with the Intercept system, which has been fully validated both in vitro and through published Phase I to IV clinical trials.[7,8] The use of these components has been being monitored through an active hemovigilance system[9,10] since 2003. Other technologies can be introduced in Belgium but need first to meet the same high standards of quality.

References

1. Van Haute L, Benoit Y, Bordon V, et al. Therapeutic efficacy and safety of transfusion of pathogen-inactivated platelets to pediatric patients. Vox Sang 2006;91(Suppl 3):177.
2. Osselear JC, Messe N, Goffaux M, et al. Validation of Intercept treatment on splitted apheresis products. Vox Sang 2004;87:269.
3. Osselaer JC, Bueno JL, Messe N, et al. Prospective active hemovigilance plan for INTERCEPT platelets in Europe: A status report. Vox Sang 2005;89(Suppl 1):248.

4. Osselaer JC, Doyen C, Graux C, et al. Prevention of transfusion-associated graft versus host disease (TA-GVHD) by photochemical treatment of platelet components: Clinical experience in routine use. Blood 2007;118(Suppl 1): 2285.
5. Osselaer JC, Doyen C, Chatelain C, et al. Impact of photochemical treatment (INTERCEPT) on platelet use in routine practice. Vox Sang 2006;91(Suppl 3):180.
6. Osselaer JC, Doyen C, Defoin L, et al. Universal adoption of pathogen inactivation of platelet components: Impact on platelet and red blood cell component use. Transfusion 2009;49:1412-22.
7. van Rhenen DJ, Gulliksson H, Cazenave JP, et al. Transfusion of pooled buffy coat platelet components prepared with photochemical pathogen inactivation treatment: The euroSPRITE trial. Blood 2003;101:2426-33.
8. McCullough J, Vesole DH, Benjamin RJ, et al. Therapeutic efficacy and safety of platelets treated with a photochemical process for pathogen inactivation: The SPRINT trial. Blood 2004;104:1534-41.
9. Osselaer JC, Cazenave JP, Lambermont M, et al. An active haemovigilance programme characterizing the safety profile of 7437 platelet transfusions prepared with amotosalen photochemical treatment. Vox Sang 2008;94:315-23.
10. Osselaer JC, Messe N, Hervig T, et al. A prospective observational cohort safety study of 5106 platelet transfusions using components prepared with photochemical pathogen inactivation treatment. Transfusion 2008;48:1061-71.

In: AuBuchon JP, Prowse CV, eds.
Pathogen Inactivation: The Penultimate Paradigm Shift
Bethesda, MD: AABB Press, 2010

14

Luxembourg: Mirasol Platelets

SIGRID CHERRIER-DE WILDE, MD

THIS CHAPTER REPORTS EXPERIENCE WITH THE Mirasol Pathogen Reduction Technology (PRT) system (CaridianBCT, Lakewood, CO) in routine daily use in the Centre Hospitalier Luxembourg, the national hospital of Luxembourg. Patients with acute leukemia and high-grade lymphomas are treated with therapies such as induction, consolidation, and intensification chemotherapy; autologous hematopoietic transplantation; and radiation therapy treatment. In addition, the hospital provides follow-up care for patients who undergo allogeneic hematopoietic transplantation in Belgium. The newly created hematology-oncology unit has 36 beds and a ca-

---

Sigrid Cherrier-De Wilde, MD, Hematologist, Department of Hematology, Centre Hospitalier Luxembourg, Luxembourg

The author has disclosed no conflicts of interest.

pacity for approximately 11,000 patient-days of hospitalization a year. About 45 to 70 patients flow through the outpatient clinic daily, with 10,000 patient visits per year. During weekends, the hospital provides another 400 ambulatory treatments annually, including transfusions, administration of antibiotics or chemotherapy, and diagnostic phlebotomies.

Blood Banking Practices in Luxembourg

The Red Cross of Luxembourg is the blood component supplier, producing Red Blood Cells, plasma, and platelet concentrates (whole-blood-derived platelets or apheresis platelets). In several surrounding countries, the production of platelet concentrates is exclusively performed by such national services of blood transfusion. Because the Red Cross of Luxembourg produces mostly platelet concentrates derived from whole blood (random pools of platelets), it is often difficult to obtain apheresis components from single donors on short notice from that supplier. Transfusion of pooled platelets often results in an increase in transfusion reactions, particularly for multiply transfused patients. These reactions include allergic reactions and a decrease in platelet count increment.

Luxembourg is unique in that blood production and transfusion can both be part of the hematology unit. This applies to our establishment, although blood components are also provided by the Red Cross. The country produces approximately half of its transfused platelet concentrates. The advantages of internal production are immediate availability, improved visibility, and simplified inventory management.

A platelet donor population is routinely defined for patients with severe hematologic diagnoses such as acute leukemia, aplastic anemia, etc, aiming for a group of about 10 dedicated donors for each specific patient. Donors are selected for a patient when the probable need for transfusion of a specific patient is identified based on a questionnaire, medical visit, and blood analysis including cell counts, biochemistry, infectious serology, and coagulation parameters. When the patient needs a transfusion of platelets, the hospital calls one of the donors from the select group and asks some additional basic questions (eg, to confirm no recent use of nonsteroidal anti-inflammatory drugs, aspirin, or other anticoagulants and no fever) before accepting a donation of apheresis platelets. (A room is dedicated to the apheresis procedures performed in the hospital, including plateletpheresis, therapeutic plasma exchange, and peripheral blood stem cell collection.) Apheresis platelets are produced in house with the aim of having the capacity to respond quickly to urgent needs for transfusion. The hospital performs bacterial screening not on individual products but only retrospectively if a transfusion reaction occurs. This allows for immediate transfusion after processing the collection. Serologic tests for infectious diseases are performed at the point of donor selection and then every 3 months. One of the measures to reduce the rate of transfusion-transmitted infection is diverting the first 15 mL of blood after skin puncture in a special vial; this amount can be used for the blood count and for adjusting the parameters of the apheresis device.

Plateletpheresis is performed on the Trima apheresis platform (CaridianBCT, Lakewood, CO). In 2009, 193 procedures were performed, resulting in about 380 single apheresis platelet units. Before implementation of the Mirasol technology, there was little control over the concentration of platelets in the apheresis bag and, more important, very limited process documentation.

Integration of Mirasol Pathogen-Reduction Technology

Overview of the Technology

In 2008, the hospital decided to test the Mirasol PRT system, mainly investigating it for ease of use of the device and adverse events in recipients. Mirasol is a safe pathogen-reduction system using a nontoxic and natural compound, riboflavin (vitamin B2). (See Fig 14-1.) It has been tested effectively against a broad range of disease-causing agents (viruses, bacteria, and parasites) and has also demonstrated inactivation of white blood cells (WBCs).[1,2] The function and viability of platelets is preserved.[3-7] The addition of riboflavin to a blood component followed by ultraviolet illumination ensures irreversible nucleotide damage to pathogens and WBCs.[8] In toxicologic studies, no toxicities from riboflavin or its photoproducts have been reported even at concentrations much higher than after full blood volume exchange in a patient.[9]

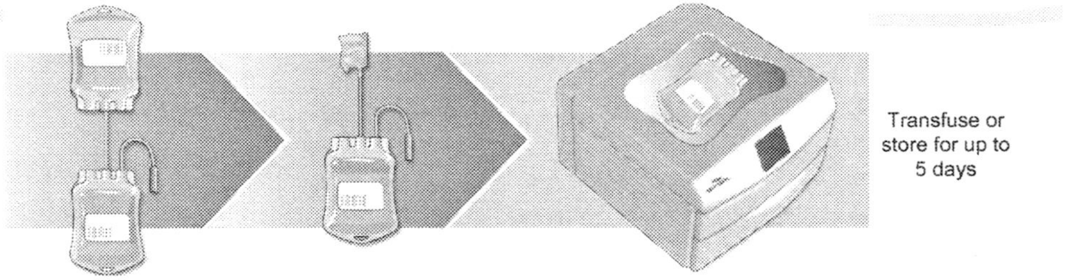

Product Requirements

Source	Apheresis (SDP) in plasma & ACD-A Buffy-coat plts (BCP) in plasma & CPD
Volume	170 - 360 mL
Concentration	0.8 - 2.1 × 10^6/μL
Yield*	Up to 7.5 × 10^{11}
Storage	0.7 - 2.1 × 10^6 platelets/μL

Process Requirements

SDP: treat within 2 - 18 hrs of collection
BCP: treat within 8 hrs of separation

CaridianBCT

*As determined by the upper treatment limits for platelet concentration and volume. PN 306690-190 ©2009 CaridianBCT

Figure 14-1. Mirasol (CaridianBCT, Lakewood, CO) process for platelets stored in plasma.
SDP = single-donor platelets; ACD-A = acid-citrate-dextrose formula A; plts = platelets; CPD = citrate-phosphate-dextrose. (Used with permission from CaridianBCT.)

The greatest transfusion risk is bacterial contamination of the platelet concentrates, and pathogen-reduction treatment reduces this risk considerably.[10] Mirasol treatment inactivates WBCs and can be used as an alternative to gamma irradiation in preventing graft-vs-host reactions after transfusion.[11] Currently, the Red Cross of Luxembourg sends blood products to Belgium or France for gamma irradiation. This has made it very difficult to produce platelets from domestic sources for patients needing irradiated labile blood components, particularly on short notice. With the implementation of pathogen-reduction technology, however, Mirasol-treated platelet concentrates can be supplied to patients who previously needed gamma-irradiated platelets. Thus the technology has enabled optimization of the donor pool while maintaining the same donor selection procedures as before implementation.

Mirasol Procedure

After apheresis collection (approximately 90 minutes), the units rest for 2 hours before further processing to allow a reduction in any aggregates that may have formed during collection. The average platelet collection volume is 260 mL per unit, and the average platelet concentration is about $1200 \times 10^3/\mu L$; contamination by red cells or leukocytes is minimal. The Mirasol procedure is rather straightforward (Fig 14-1). First, there is the transfer of the platelets from the collection bag to a special bag used for illumination and storage. The estimated loss in transfer is less than 3 mL. Replacement of the current Trima bag with the Mirasol illumination and storage bag could significantly reduce both the cost and the complexity of the process even further, and CaridianBCT is currently developing this capacity (R. Goodrich, personal communication). Elimination of the transfer could reduce both the time required for the nurse and the contamination risk correlated with this product transfer. The second step is the addition of riboflavin to the platelet concentrate via a sterile connection device. All air remaining in the final mixture is manually purged into the empty riboflavin bag, which is then discarded. Before measuring the final weight of the unit, all remaining tubes are sealed so that it is a completely closed bag. In routine operation, these pre-illumination steps require about 5 minutes. Using the final weight of the bag, the Mirasol device calculates the exact time for the illumination, which ranges between 6 and 10 minutes.

Directly after illumination, the treated platelet unit is ready for transfusion or for storage in a standard platelet agitator.

The software built into Mirasol systems is a simple, intuitive software program to provide efficient data management and reporting. All unit and reagent data are scanned to avoid errors associated with manual data transcription. In addition, the software prevents the repeat illumination of previously treated units and prints labels to identify units that have been successfully illuminated. These steps provide a complete overview of every unit treated (lot and kit number), including the donor information, the content, and the destination. At present this information is saved as a paper file, but it will later be integrated into the hospital's electronic system, allowing access to all laboratory and illumination results in one location. (Before 2008, this information was recorded manually in each patient file; the automated traceability now meets common standards.)

Costs

Costs for implementing the system have been substantial, but the facility has decided to proceed in the interest of improved patient safety and health benefits. The risk reduction for bacterial contamination, viral infections, unknown pathogens, and WBC-mediated transfusion events were drivers for introduction of this technology. The short processing times of the Mirasol PRT system were also viewed as very manageable in the actual work flow. Finally, the reduction in costs by eliminating gamma irradiation provided some cost mitigation and was a major advantage that factored into the decision-making process.

Implementation

In the spring of 2008, during the validation study with the Mirasol system, 60 procedures were performed without any problems. The data in this initial evaluation was obtained by monitoring in-vitro product characteristics, production times, and ease-of-use parameters. Results were consistent with those reported previously in studies conducted in over 19 locations in seven separate countries in Europe as part of the Mirasol Evaluation Program (see Tables 14-1 through 14-3).[12]

Table 14-1. Mirasol Evaluation Program Study Design*

Countries Participating	Collection Platforms	Number of Products Treated	Number of Products Transfused
Spain, Italy, Poland, Turkey, Portugal, Lithuania, and Luxembourg (19 locations)	Orbisac[†] Manual buffy-coat (4- and 5-unit pools) Trima Accel[†] Amicus[‡] Haemonetics[§] MCS+	444	246

*Used with permission from CaridianBCT; see also Marschner et al.[12]
[†]CaridianBCT, Lakewood, CO.
[‡]Fenwal, Lake Zurich, IL.
[§]Haemonetics, Braintree, MA.

Table 14-2. In-Vitro Cell Quality Parameters from Mirasol Evaluation Program Studies*

	Before Illumination	After Illumination	Day 5 of Storage
Number of units	204	138	98
pH (22 C)	7.24 ±0.16	7.21 ±0.15	6.99 ±0.21
Swirl	3 ±0	3 ±0	2.6 ±0.5
Yield	3.5 ±0.5	3.4 ±0.5	3.2 ±0.7

*Used with permission from CaridianBCT; see also Marschner et al.[12]

Table 14-3. Mirasol Process Assessment from Mirasol Evaluation Program Studies*

	Processing Time	Ease-of-Use Rating†	Rating of Integration into Current Workflow†
Bag transfer	6.6 ±3.8 minutes	3.75	
Illumination	6.1 ±2.0 minutes	4	3.75
Overall	12.7 ±4.2 minutes	4	
Number of units or sites	99 units	4 sites	4 sites

*Used with permission from CaridianBCT; see also Marschner et al.[12]
†Excellent score = 4; poor score = 1.

In June 2009, routine Mirasol treatment was implemented for all apheresis platelet units. As of the end of June 2010, the hospital had performed 520 procedures, providing treated platelets for about 25 patients, with a donor pool of 200 individuals.

Continuing Evaluation

The facility is currently participating in a postmarket surveillance study—a single-center, observational, postapproval study (PROWESS). The parameters being evaluated in this study include incidence of serious adverse events, 1-hour and 24-hour corrected platelet count increments (CCIs), incidence of (World Health Organization) Grade 3 and 4 bleeding events, and intervals between platelet and red cell transfusions. Results from a preliminary analysis of the data in these patients are consistent with prior publications and observations reported by others in the field (Table 14-4). The observed posttransfusion increment of platelet count is heterogeneous and a function of the patient's pathology and clinical status. So far, no increase has been observed in either platelet or red cell use after implementation of Mirasol PRT. CCI values at 1 hour have been around 10,000 on average for stable patients with hematologic malignancies. All transfusions monitored to date (n = 30) have demonstrated a positive CCI at 1 hour, and 63% of those have demonstrated values 7500 at 1 hour, a value commonly used to define a "successful" transfusion. These values are in agreement with those reported in the randomized, prospective clinical trial conducted with the Mirasol product in France (MIRACLE Trial).[13] The hospital intends to continue data collection in this study format and to present results in 2011.

Adverse Events

Observations regarding adverse events associated with transfusion have also been consistent with prior reports from surveillance and hemovigilance reporting at five sites routinely using the Mirasol product. A total of 3803 transfusions were tracked in eight countries, and seven adverse events related to transfusion were reported (0.2%). Luxembourg observed one patient who reacted twice to Mirasol-treated platelets. The patient reacted to both units from a

Table 14-4. Transfusion Outcomes of Mirasol-Treated Platelets

Data Source	Product Type	Storage Solution	Average 1-Hour CCI	Average 24-Hour CCI
MIRACLE study[13]	Apheresis and pooled buffy coat	Plasma	11,725	6676
Site 1,[14] Mirasol Evaluation Program	Orbisac buffy coat	Plasma	ND	6351
Site 2, PROWESS study (unpublished data*)	Manual buffy coat	Plasma	ND	5185

*Submitted to *TRANSFUSION* abstract supplement (2010).
CCI = correct count increment; ND = not determined.

double apheresis collection with moderate erythema of the skin. The patient did not further react to any other Mirasol-treated platelet units from other donors. These results suggested that the two reactions were the result of an incompatibility between donor and recipient rather than associated with the Mirasol process specifically.

Before implementation of Mirasol-treated platelets, prophylactic treatment with anti-histamines and corticosteroids was occasionally required with some patients before transfusion to avoid transfusion reactions. Since implementation, the number of patients requiring this prophylactic treatment has dramatically decreased, along with the frequency of observed transfusion reactions. The hospital intends to perform a prospective study to document an observed reduction in the use of antihistamines and corticosteroids, although logistical issues at this site may make such a controlled study difficult to implement.

Conclusion

In conclusion, the hospital is very satisfied with the production of platelet concentrates using the Mirasol system for platelets. The process provides several advantages:

- Apheresis procedures coupled with a simple pathogen-reduction procedure that does not introduce toxicology concerns for either the staff or the patients who come in contact with the product.
- Software to capture and summarize all data related to the unit (donor, patient, concentration of platelets, container identification, etc).
- Increased safety of platelet transfusions for patients, with an observed reduction in prophylactic use of drugs intended to reduce allergic reactions.
- No time-consuming procedures for personnel, and rapid release of the units after processing.
- Ability to provide a platelet unit with performance equivalent to gamma-irradiated units in a much more feasible and practical way than could be achieved previously.

References

1. Fast LD, DiLeone G, Li J, Goodrich R. Functional inactivation of white blood cells by Mirasol treatment. Transfusion 2006;46:642-8.
2. Ruane PH, Edrich R, Gampp D, et al. Photochemical inactivation of selected viruses and bacteria in platelet concentrates using riboflavin and light. Transfusion 2004;44:877-85.
3. Li J, de Korte D, Woolum MD, et al. Pathogen reduction of buffy coat platelet concentrates using riboflavin and light: Comparisons with pathogen-reduction technology-treated apheresis platelet products. Vox Sang 2004;87:82-90.
4. Li J, Goodrich L, Hansen E, et al. Platelet glycolytic flux increases stimulated by ultraviolet-induced stress is not the direct cause of platelet morphology and activation changes: Possible implications for the role of glucose in platelet storage. Transfusion 2005;45:1750-8.
5. Li J, Lockerbie O, de Korte D, et al. Evaluation of platelet mitochondria integrity after treatment with Mirasol pathogen reduction technology. Transfusion 2005;45:920-6.
6. Picker SM, Steisel A, Gathof BS. Effects of Mirasol PRT treatment on storage lesion development in plasma-stored apheresis-derived platelets compared to untreated and irradiated units. Transfusion 2008;48:1685-92.
7. Picker SM. Cell integrity and mitochondrial function after Mirasol-PRT treatment for pathogen reduction of apheresis-derived platelets: Results of a 3-arm in vitro study. Transfus Apher Sci 2009;40:79-85.
8. Kumar V, Lockerbie O, Keil SD, et al. Riboflavin and UV-light based pathogen reduction: Extent and consequence of DNA damage at the molecular level. Photochem Photobiol 2004;80:15-21.
9. Reddy HL, Dayan AD, Cavagnaro J, et al. Toxicity testing of a novel riboflavin-based technology for pathogen reduction and white blood cell inactivation. Transfus Med Rev 2008;22:133-53.
10. Goodrich RP, Gilmour D, Hovenga N, Keil SD. A laboratory comparison of pathogen reduction technology treatment and culture of platelet products for addressing bacterial contamination concerns. Transfusion 2009;49:1205-16.
11. Fast LD, DiLeone G, Cardarelli G, et al. Mirasol PRT treatment of donor white blood cells prevents the development of xenogeneic graft-versus-host disease in Rag2-/-gamma c-/- double knockout mice. Transfusion 2006;46: 1553-60.
12. Marschner S, Villaescusa RD, Perez Vaquero MA, et al. The Mirasol Evaluation Program: Use of Mirasol pathogen reduction technology for platelets in routine clinical practice. Vox Sang 2009;96(Suppl 1):229.
13. The Mirasol Clinical Evaluation Study Group. A randomized controlled clinical trial evaluating the performance and safety of platelets treated with MIRASOL pathogen reduction technology. Transfusion 2010 May 18 (epub ahead of print)
14. Blanco L, Yanez M, Gonzalez A, et al. Performance of buffy coat platelets in plasma treated with riboflavin and UV light: In-vitro and in-vivo evaluation (abstract). Transfusion 2009;49(Suppl):84A.

In: AuBuchon JP, Prowse CV, eds.
Pathogen Inactivation: The Penultimate Paradigm Shift
Bethesda, MD: AABB Press, 2010

15

United States: Solvent/ Detergent Plasma

BERNARD HOROWITZ, PhD

SOLVENT/DETERGENT-TREATED PLASMA (SD PLASMA) was conceived by this author in 1986 or 1987 with the primary goal of eliminating the transmission of hepatitis B virus (HBV); non-A,non-B hepatitis virus (NANBHV); and human immunodeficiency virus (HIV) by Fresh Frozen Plasma (FFP) and other single-donor blood plasma products. At that time, successful implementation of SD plasma would mean prevention of the transmission of several hundred cases of HBV and AIDS and 10,000 cases of NANBHV. It was reasonable to believe that SD treatment of plasma could achieve this goal because the author and many collaborating scientists and phy-

Bernard Horowitz, PhD, Horowitz Consultants, LLC, Key Biscayne, Florida

The author has disclosed a financial relationship with New York Blood Center.

sicians had already shown that SD treatment applied to coagulation factor concentrates killed these viruses quickly and completely while leaving intact the labile coagulation factors that were needed in therapy. A secondary objective was to convert FFP from a highly variable single-donor product with unit-to-unit two- or threefold differences in coagulation factor content to a pharmaceutical product akin to other purified plasma products prepared by plasma fractionators worldwide. The product would be sterile filtered, cell free, and low in particulates and have consistent levels of coagulation factors and guaranteed presence of a variety of antibodies, including antibodies to parvovirus B19 and hepatitis A virus (HAV).

SD plasma was introduced first in Europe in the early 1990s and was licensed by the Food and Drug Administration (FDA) in 1998. Before licensure by the FDA, the potential availability in the United States of this safer substitute for FFP stimulated great debate, at times over scientific or medical concerns and at times over rising health-care costs and the potential loss of blood center and blood bank revenues. The availability of SD plasma in the United States ceased only several years after its introduction.

This chapter describes some of the salient events that delayed the US introduction of SD plasma and that led to its ultimate rejection by the blood banking community. The status of SD plasma at the time of licensure by the FDA has been published[1] and will not be repeated here. In short, this is more akin to a view from the board room than one from the bedside or the laboratory bench. Some of this experience may apply to newer attempts to provide virally inactivated blood components in the United States and elsewhere.

Collaboration with Octapharma and European Adoption and Utilization

In 1986-1987 the author applied to the New York Blood Center (NYBC, his employer) for funds to cover the initial laboratory development for SD plasma and, despite initial encouragement, was turned down after an individual at the FDA unofficially indicated that, given the overuse of FFP, it would be better to de-license FFP than license a safer alternative. Consequently, this author approached Wolfgang Marguerre and Robert Taub of Octapharma to assess their interest. At that time, Octapharma was working closely with several European blood centers and had adopted SD treatment for its coagulation factor concentrates. NYBC accepted Octapharma's offer to fund the laboratory development effort in exchange for Octapharma's receiving European marketing rights. Principally with the assistance of Richard Bonomo, the laboratory development effort was completed in 1989, one year from initiation.

As compared with SD treatment of purified blood derivatives and based on marker virus kill studies, the concentration of tri-n-butyl phosphate (TNBP) was raised from 0.3% to 1% to accommodate plasma's lipid content, and the temperature was raised to 30 C to ensure rapid and vigorous virus kill.[2] Triton X-100 was selected as the detergent because Bonomo showed that it and TNBP could be removed by a simple but effective hydrophobic chromatography step.[3] Subsequently, removal of the SD reagents by hydrophobic chromatography was very useful in the preparation of other products. Before this chromatographic step, the SD and plasma mixture was extracted with soybean oil, a procedure first developed by Drs. Kenneth Woods and Thomas Orme to overcome column poisoning when processing antihemophilic factor concentrate with TNBP/cholate.[4]

This laboratory process was transferred to Octapharma which—working with the Red Cross center in Hagen, Germany—transformed it into a full manufacturing process. Because of the way blood components were regulated in Germany, SD plasma entered routine clinical use in the German federal state of North Rhine Westphalia in 1991. In 1992 Norway decided to fully replace FFP with SD plasma [termed Octaplas (Octapharma AG, Lachen, Switzerland)] nationwide based on initial clinical trial data (since greatly extended[5]) and its perceived viral safety advantage. Shortly thereafter, SD plasma totally replaced FFP in Belgium and was also in routine use in both France and Germany. Simultaneously, toxicology studies sponsored by Octapharma and viral kill studies of HBV and hepatitis C virus (HCV) in the chimpanzee model performed at NYBC by this author's laboratory in collaboration with Alfred Prince were completed. From the initial availability of SD plasma through 2009, Octapharma in its factory in Austria together with its European licensees in Hagen, Germany and Bordeaux, France distributed approximately 10 million units of SD plasma for use in routine medical care. There have been no documented cases of transmission of HBV, HCV, or HIV—a record no single-donor blood product can claim.

US Manufacture and Clinical Trials

By 1990-1991 it became clear that the FDA's attitude toward a safer form of FFP had changed, possibly because it received feedback from clinicians who expressed the viewpoint that FFP was an essential product and that a safer form would be welcome, and possibly because the transmission of NANBHV (now renamed HCV) continued despite the discovery by the Chiron group of the causative viral agent and the development and deployment of specific, serologic tests. Melville Biologics (a division of NYBC) began manufacturing SD plasma in 1991-92 using many of the same procedures implemented at Hagen and initiated clinical studies under an investigational new drug (IND) application approved by the FDA. These trials were led by Drs. Marilyn Horowitz and Joan Pehta at NYBC and eventually by Drs. Howard Grossberg and Joan Pehta as part of V.I. Technologies, Inc, abbreviated as VITEX. (VITEX was formed because NYBC lacked adequate resources to pursue SD plasma and a number of other product-related opportunities.)

Because FFP itself had never undergone federal licensing trials, the clinical trials needed for licensure for SD plasma were unknown. Consequently, multiple clinical trials were initiated, with most using FFP as the control: one in patients with congenital, single coagulation factor deficiencies (Factor V, Factor XI, Factor XIII, and fibrinogen); one in liver disease patients with multiple coagulation factor deficiencies; one in warfarin reversal where the so-called vitamin-K-dependent coagulation factors needed to be restored rapidly; and one in patients with chronic, relapsing thrombotic thrombocytopenic purpura (TTP), expanded to include acute TTP once efficacy was demonstrated in the former. Each of the studies concluded that SD plasma was both safe and efficacious and, when FFP was used as the control, equivalent to FFP.[5-10] SD plasma was reported to have fewer adverse events associated with its use than did FFP in the treatment of TTP,[11] likely because the processing of SD plasma removed large quantities of lipids and cellular debris and because of the large volumes administered when treating this disorder. Additionally, no episodes of transfusion-related acute lung injury (TRALI) were observed despite infusion of 4000 units of SD plasma into over 150 patients.

Licensure in the United States

As clinical data accumulated and were published, a significant sector of the US blood banking community expressed concern over the licensure of SD plasma. To expand the dialog and receive feedback, in 1995 the National Institutes of Health and the FDA jointly sponsored a workshop titled "The Role of Virally Inactivated Plasma in Transfusion Medicine." This general title was required because neither group could sponsor a workshop on a specific product, even though SD plasma was the only product discussed. Presentations included evidence of viral safety, data from manufacture at VITEX, toxicology data developed under Octapharma sponsorship, and clinical safety and efficacy data from both the United States and Europe. These data made clear that US licensure of SD plasma was justified. The single largest concern voiced by the audience related to availability. In supplying hospitals, blood centers did not want to compete with one another based on which center had SD plasma and which did not, and they also were reluctant to maintain two inventories, one of FFP and one of the "safer" alternative. The "take-home message" was clear: before VITEX launched SD plasma and the FDA licensed it, capacity for the manufacture of 2,000,000 units/year had to be in place. At the time, VITEX could manufacture approximately 500,000 units/year. Additional voiced concerns related to the cost of the new product and the possibility that, because of pooling, the transmission of an unknown, nonenveloped virus might be more widespread than would occur with single-donor blood products. One audience member advanced a new thought, namely that because SD plasma was pooled, perhaps the best reason for its use was that it would reduce the incidence of TRALI.

As a result of this meeting, VITEX increased its manufacturing capacity over the next 18 to 24 months. In December 1996, the Blood Products Advisory Committee to the FDA recommended licensure, and VITEX's biologics license application was approved May 6, 1998, 5 years following its initial filing. The licensed indications were 1) for use in the treatment of patients with documented deficiencies of coagulation factors for which there are no concentrate preparations available, including congenital single-factor deficiencies of Factors I, V, VII, XI, and XIII and acquired multiple coagulation factor deficiencies; 2) treatment for reversals of warfarin effect; and 3) treatment of patients with TTP. The salient features of SD plasma and its manufacture are summarized in Table 15-1. Some of these features differ markedly from other pathogen-inactivated plasma replacement products in clinical use or under development.

Table 15-1. Features of SD Plasma

Inactivation chemistry

Chemicals: TNBP and Triton X-100

Mechanism of action: Extraction of viral lipids; noncovalent chemistry

Chemical residue following removal: ≤3 ppm (≥99.97% removal); no breakdown products

Pathogen elimination

≥6 $\log_{10}$ evidenced inactivation plus a high reserve capacity (see Horowitz/Busch[12] for definition)

Nonenveloped viruses: Not inactivated; viral neutralization possible; as of 1999, tested for parovirus B19 DNA

Bacteria and parasites: Removed via sterile filtration

Other aspects of manufacture

Number of units pooled: ≤2500

Sterile filtered (0.2 µ)

Multiple in-process controls, including assessment of inactivation chemicals

Full quality control release

100% visual inspection of all manufactured units for particles

Full quality assurance oversight

Product characteristics

Uniform composition

Normal or near normal procoagulant activities and most other proteins

Protein S, protein C, and anti-plasmin levels reduced

Large vWF multimers missing

Guaranteed presence of anti-parvovirus and anti-HAV

Intact cells absent and cellular debris greatly reduced

Blood center requirements

Little impact on operations, staffing, or space requirements

TNBP = tri-n-butyl phosphate; vWF = von Willebrand factor; HAV = hepatitis A virus.

Market Introduction

In the months before licensure, the FDA asked to review VITEX's product distribution plan, requesting details about how product would be moved from the VITEX warehouse to secondary distribution points and then onto blood centers and hospitals—all assuming that VITEX would need to provide the nation with 2,000,000 units of SD plasma annually. VITEX believed that its own facilities could handle the initial distribution and that it would engage outside warehousing as the demand warranted. This answer did not satisfy the FDA, and licensure was delayed. What appeared to be a stalemate to VITEX was broken only after VITEX agreed to let the American Red Cross (ARC) handle distribution; however, this agreement came at high cost. The ARC would supply all of the plasma to be processed into SD plasma, would be the exclusive US distributor, would be responsible for branding the product, and would set the price. The product would carry the ARC logo. VITEX would manufacture and comarket the product. Non-Red-Cross centers, essentially all members of America's Blood Centers, expressed dissatisfaction with this arrangement. They are responsible for collecting and distributing half of the nation's blood supply, and although all were guaranteed access to the product, the question remained as to what would happen to the plasma they would normally distribute as FFP, and there were objections to distributing product with the ARC logo because, in many cases, the ARC was a competitor. Furthermore, the ARC set the price 30% higher than expected. Thus, the intended market for the product was not responsive.

Nonenveloped Viruses

In 1986-87, when first contemplating the product, the author met with Bernard Cohen, one of the world's leading experts on parvovirus B19, to better understand the virus's biology and the risk or risks it posed. Cohen expressed surprise that anyone would be concerned. Half of the population was immune, antibody was neutralizing, and except for pregnant women, infections were generally asymptomatic or very mild and self-limiting. Nonetheless, on licensure, the FDA required VITEX to conduct a Phase IV clinical trial designed to assess parvovirus B19 and HAV transmission. The trial, designed by Grossberg and Pehta, enrolled normal volunteers who lacked antibodies to parvovirus B19 and HAV. Each received 1 unit (200 mL) of SD plasma, and serum samples were monitored for viral nucleic acid before, immediately following, and at designated times after infusion. The results were correlated with subsequently measured viral nucleic acid levels in the product. The results from the Phase IV trial were both surprising and clear-cut: when parvovirus B19 DNA exceeded 10^7 genome equivalents/mL (GE/mL), virus replication was evident, in many subjects lasting 6 months or more. Although mostly asymptomatic, infection was persistent. When parvovirus B19 DNA was 10^4 GE/mL or less, there was no evidence of viral replication; ie, the copresence of antibody was sufficient to prevent or limit infection.[13] Based on these results, VITEX recalled over 30 lots of product that had already been distributed, and instituted routine parvovirus B19 testing of minipools, setting a cutoff of 10^4 GE/mL. This specification has since been adopted by regulatory bodies and fractionators worldwide for purified blood derivatives. The clinical trial found no evidence of HAV replication. This experience demonstrates the importance of the FDA requirement for Phase IV trials and the benefit of conducting them expeditiously.

Market Withdrawal

Although the two factors described above (US marketing issues and threats from nonenveloped viruses) might have forced VITEX to discontinue manufacture, an additional finding needs to be mentioned. One of the intended uses of SD plasma was in the treatment of liver transplant patients, who generally require coagulation factor supplementation via plasma transfusions. Although SD plasma has been used successfully by others in this setting,[14] Cedars Sinai Medical Center (Los Angeles) reported six deaths among 31 or 32 patients caused by unwanted thrombosis that was ascribed to SD plasma. Although investigations failed to establish a cause-and-effect relationship, this possibility is supported by the laboratory finding that SD plasma had low levels of protein S and protein C. Thromboembolic complications have not generally been associated with the use of Octaplas (the European product), and further analysis revealed that although the US product was manufactured by similar (though not identical) methods, the anticoagulant content of Octaplas was higher.[15,16] To this author's knowledge, the processing step(s) that caused this difference have not been identified but could involve the quality of the input plasma.[17] To the disappointment of at least some physicians whose clinical experience with the product was positive, manufacture of the US product ceased in 2002-2003.

Conclusions and Possible Lessons Learned

From the scientific perspective, the experience with SD plasma demonstrates the difficulty in re-engineering a traditional blood component. Unlike other viral-inactivation approaches applied to blood components, the SD treatment functions via a noncovalent chemistry that inherently is nondestructive to most protein structures. Moreover, SD treatments had already been applied successfully to purified blood derivatives, including proteins considered to be quite labile. Nonetheless, plasma is a complex fluid, and, to the detriment of select patient groups, it is possible that the required balance between procoagulant and anticoagulant activities was not adequately maintained by the form of SD plasma prepared at VITEX. Pathogen inactivation of red cell and platelet concentrates presents an even greater challenge. Cells are inherently more complex than proteins, and because these concentrates contain multiple cell types as well as plasma, the covalent chemistries that are being explored raise the possibility that any of the constituents might be functionally compromised or become immunogenic as a result of treatment.

An equally important conclusion is that it is difficult to make fundamental changes to blood banking practices. Transfusion specialists are most comfortable using donor selection and donor screening to achieve safety. When new pathogen threats arise, blood banking specialists study and report on them, and—when necessary, available, and convenient—deploy new tests for them. Safety is improved incrementally over time, with tests added pathogen-by-pathogen and with improved versions of tests replacing earlier versions. This approach has two distinct advantages, namely that new safety measures apply equally to all blood components and that no matter how many tests are run, the product to be transfused is not compromised.

Most people in the transfusion community acknowledge that pathogen inactivation is conceptually the superior approach.[18] It can provide large safety margins, it addresses the window period in a way that no testing can, it attacks mutants not detected by current test methodology, and it eliminates viruses and other pathogens for which there are no tests. It also accommodates laboratory error, though a rare occurrence. Despite these considerations and its broad acceptance in other fields, pathogen inactivation appears to pose a conceptual hurdle to many blood banking specialists. There appears to be greater comfort with the continuous threat of pathogens contaminating blood products than with the uncertainties engendered by pathogen inactivation. In the case of SD plasma, the possibility that pooling might increase risk of nonenveloped virus transmission was a common concern, but seldom mentioned were the advantages of processing in a true manufacturing facility using proven methods and disciplines developed by blood plasma fractionators over decades (uniform product, sterile filtration, lot release with full quality control, extremely efficient removal of process chemicals, significant reduction of cellular debris, and guaranteed presence of a broad spectrum of antibodies, including viral antibodies).

A third conclusion relates to timing. What may be a compelling story in one decade may become far less compelling in the face of subsequent advances. When this author first considered applying SD treatment to FFP, substitution of SD plasma for FFP would have prevented exposures of approximately 10,000 patients/year to one of the three principal viruses of concern in a plasma transfusion setting—ie, HBV, HCV, or HIV. By 1993, following the availability of anti-HCV screening tests and when NYBC first submitted its license application for SD plasma, this number had dropped to 52 patients/year,[19] and today SD plasma would prevent exposure to one of these three viruses in fewer than 10 patients annually.[20,21] Nonetheless, as summarized well by Dr. Harvey Alter, had pathogen-inactivation systems been in place when West Nile virus outbreaks first occurred in the United States in 1999, none of the 4480 projected transfusion-transmitted transmissions would have occurred.[18] This message is amplified further by Stramer et al, who cataloged 63 infectious agents potentially transmissible by blood, most of which do not have an available intervention strategy that would prevent transmission by transfusion.[22]

So, what of the US experience with SD plasma can be applied to the US introduction of pathogen-inactivated blood concentrates prepared by alternative chemistries? Only time will tell, but what is clear is that many of the criticisms raised in the 1990s are applicable today. The products are likely to be costly; the safety advantage of a pathogen-inactivated component will be diluted when a patient also receives other blood components not available in a pathogen-inactivated form; maintaining two product inventories, one treated to inactivate pathogens and the other untreated, is confusing to patients and to many practicing physicians; and inevitably there will be questions of safety arising from measurable changes in the blood product and from adverse events in patients, where it is very difficult to determine causal relationships. Moreover, some hurdles today are even higher. On the one hand, as a consequence of improved testing, blood truly is safer than when the work on SD plasma first began or even when it was first licensed, and the development cycle for new tests has been greatly shortened. On the other hand, the ever increasing number of blood-borne pathogens detected by improved monitoring systems worldwide, together with more extensive travel, favor the adoption of broad-spectrum pathogen inactivation. This author hopes that the technology and the transfusion community are up to the challenge.

References

1. Klein HG, Dodd RY, Dzik WH, et al. Current status of solvent/detergent-treated frozen plasma. Transfusion 1998;38:102-7.
2. Horowitz B, Bonomo R, Prince AM, et al. Solvent/detergent-treated plasma: A virus-inactivated substitute for fresh frozen plasma. Blood 1992;79:826-31.
3. Bonomo RJ. Removal of process chemicals from labile biological mixtures by hydrophobic interaction chromatography. US Patent 5,094,960. Washington, DC: US Patent Office, 1992.
4. Woods KR, Orme TW. Removal of lipid soluble process chemicals from biological materials by extraction with naturally occurring oils or synthetic substitutes thereof. US Patent 4,789,545, 1988.
5. Solheim BG, Rollag H, Svennevig JL, et al. Viral safety of solvent/detergent-treated plasma. Transfusion 2000;40:84-90.
6. Pehta JC, Sellers PW, Horowitz MS, SD Plasma Study Group. Clinical studies with SD plasma in patients with factor deficiencies. Thromb Haemost 1993; 69:808.

7. Chintagumpala M, Moake J, Turner N, et al. Transfusion with fresh-frozen plasma or solvent/detergent-treated plasma reverses both thrombocytopenia and excessive von Willebrand factor-mediated shear-induced platelet aggregation in chronic relapsing thrombotic thrombocytopenic purpura (TTP) (abstract). Blood 1992;80(Suppl 1):63a.
8. Moake J, Chintagumpala M, Turner N, et al. Solvent/detergent-treated plasma suppresses shear-induced platelet aggregation and prevents episodes of thrombotic thrombocytopenic purpura. Blood 1994;84:490-7.
9. Horowitz MS, Pehta JC. SD Plasma in TTP and coagulation factor deficiencies for which no concentrates are available. Vox Sang 1998;74(Suppl 1): 231-5.
10. Lerner RG, Nelson J, Sorcia E, et al. Evaluation of solvent/detergent-treated plasma in patients with a prolonged prothrombin time. Vox Sang 2000;79: 161-7.
11. McCarthy LJ. Evidence-based medicine for apheresis: An ongoing challenge. Ther Apher Dial 2004;8:112-23.
12. Horowitz B, Busch M. Estimating the pathogen safety of manufactured human plasma products: Application to fibrin sealants and to thrombin. Transfusion 2008;48:1739-53.
13. Brown KE, Young NS, Alving BM, Barbosa LH. Parvovirus B19: Implications for transfusion medicine. Summary of a workshop (see comments by J. Pehta). Transfusion 2001;41:130-5.
14. Williamson LM, Llewelyn CA, Fisher NC, et al. A randomized trial of solvent/ detergent-treated and standard fresh frozen plasma in the coagulopathy of liver disease and liver transplantation. Transfusion 2009;39:1227-34.
15. Beeck H, Hellstern P. In vitro characterization of solvent/detergent-treated human plasma and of quarantine fresh frozen plasma. Vox Sang 1998;74 (Suppl 1):219-23.
16. Salge-Bartels U, Breitner-Ruddock S, Hunfeld A, et al. Are quality differences responsible for different adverse reactions reported for SD plasma from USA and Europe? Transfus Med 2006;16:266-75.
17. Magner JJ, Crowley KJ, Boylan JF, et al. Fatal fibrinolysis during orthotopic liver transplantation in patients receiving solvent/detergent-treated plasma (Octaplas). J Cardiothorac Vasc Anesth 2007;21:410-13.
18. Alter HJ. Pathogen reduction: A precautionary principle paradigm. Transfus Med Rev 2008;22:97-102.
19. Schreiber GB, Busch MP, Kleinman SH, Korelitz JJ. The risk of transfusion-transmitted viral infections. The Retrovirus Epidemiology Donor Study. N Engl J Med 1996;334:1685-90.
20. Stramer SL. Current risks of transfusion-transmitted agents: A review. Arch Pathol Lab Med 2007;13:702-7.
21. Zou S, Stramer SL, Notari EP, et al. Current incidence and residual risk of hepatitis B infection among blood donors in the United States. Transfusion 2009;49:1609-20.
22. Stramer SL, Hollinger FB, Katz LM, et al. Emerging infectious disease agents and their potential threat to transfusion safety. Transfusion 2009;49(Suppl 2):1S-29S.

In: AuBuchon JP, Prowse CV, eds.
Pathogen Inactivation: The Penultimate Paradigm Shift
Bethesda, MD: AABB Press, 2010

16

US Perspectives on Implementation

LOUIS M. KATZ, MD, AND CELSO BIANCO, MD

Unfortunately, the balance of nature decrees that a superabundance of dreams is paid for by a growing potential for nightmares.

—Peter Ustinov

THE DRIVER OF THE TRANSFUSION MEDICINE COMMUNITY toward pathogen inactivation (PI) is recipient safety. Most of this volume reports the basic science and clinical research that supports the clinical advantages of PI:

- The inactivation of viruses, bacteria, and parasites that may be transmitted from donors will protect recipients. For susceptible agents, this includes their infectious "window periods" during which they may escape detection by current donor recruitment, interviewing, examination, and testing methods.

Louis M. Katz, MD, Executive Vice President, Medical Affairs, Mississippi Valley Regional Blood Center, Davenport, Iowa, and Celso Bianco, MD, Executive Vice President, America's Blood Centers, Washington, District of Columbia

L. Katz has disclosed financial relationships with Abbott Diagnostics, Chiron Corporation, Roche Molecular Systems, and Ortho Clinical Diagnostics. C. Bianco has disclosed no conflicts of interest.

- Inactivation of the transfused white blood cells responsible for transfusion-associated graft-vs-host disease (TA-GVHD) may well render obsolete the use of blood irradiators that require clinicians to recognize recipients at risk and present important safety, logistic, and security issues to collection facilities and transfusion services.
- In addition to protecting recipients, implementation of PI should allow the transfusion medicine community to reconsider how donor history deferrals and donor screening assays are used—not only for infections currently addressed but also, probably more important given contemporary levels of transfusion safety from infectious agents, for those to which the community will inevitably be *reacting* in the future.
- To the degree that white cells are inactivated in cellular components and plasma is diluted or replaced by additive solutions during PI, there may be other advantages. These include prevention of febrile reactions and alloimmunization and mitigation of tranfusion-related acute lung injury (TRALI) if levels of viable leukocytes, pathogenic antibodies, and/or other biologic response modifiers are sufficiently reduced in transfusion products. These potential benefits are yet to be demonstrated and quantified in robust clinical studies.

Transfusion-Transmitted Pathogens

The utility of preventing transfusion transmission of known pathogens is evident. Candidate PI systems are robust against the agents involved in the recent epidemics of transfusion-transmitted human immunodeficiency virus (HIV) and hepatitis C virus (HCV) that were associated with enormous morbidity and mortality. It is important to recall that in San Francisco early during the AIDS epidemic, 1% of donations were given by individuals infected with HIV.[1]

Bacteria

Bacterial contamination of blood components, especially platelets stored at room temperature, is associated with more deaths than all other infectious risks combined.[2] Current estimates of the incidence of platelet-associated sepsis range as high as 1/1000 therapeutic doses transfused, with a *fatality* rate of 10 to 20/1,000,000 units.[3-6] The approaches to mitigation include straightforward donor acceptability criteria, effective arm inspection and skin preparation techniques, and diversion from the collection bag of the initial aliquot of donor blood with the bacteria-rich dermal plug that it can contain. A variety of surrogate measures, including visual examination for platelet swirling, pH and glucose measurements, and bacterial staining with microscopic examination, have been used to predict the presence of clinically significant contamination but are insufficiently sensitive and specific. Quality control testing using culture-based methods has been widely implemented and, most recently, the option to test platelets late in storage with point-of-release tests for the presence of bacteria has become available. Despite these interventions, only about half of bacterially contaminated products may be interdicted, and septic reactions and deaths are still recognized when detection is prevented by low numbers of bacteria present during the early hours of storage and by the limited volume of a component that can be sampled for culture.[7-9] Residual risk from bacteria recently resulted in the early termination of the PASSPORT study of the safety of 7-day dating for apheresis platelets—an action that some believe could actually have resulted in a net decrease in the safety of platelet transfusion, amid complex circumstances, by causing a delay in the implementation of TRALI mitigation strategies.[10]

All of the PI methods being developed for platelet components inactivate levels of relevant bacteria that are orders of magnitude higher than those present early after collection, when PI will be applied. In addition to the safety increment from inactivation of bacteria, if cultures can be discontinued [as in some areas of the European Union (EU) after adoption of PI], it will result in extra availability for platelets at the hospital because they can be distributed without the delay required before culture inoculation and for incubation. A return in the United States to 7-day (or longer) apheresis platelet dating might be considered if in-vitro function, recovery, and survival of PI platelets are adequate.[11]

Parasites

Babesiosis, an erythrocyte infection caused by *Babesia microti* and related species in the United States, is a conundrum. Transfusion transmission has been documented since 1968.[12] Transmissions and deaths are well recognized and believed to be both underreported and increasing.[13] Donor history questions have poor positive and negative predictive values for identifying infected donors,[14] dampening enthusiasm for their use in interventions to prevent transfusion transmission of *Babesia sp.* Moreover, the restricted, if expanding, geographic distribution of the risk for infection does not generate enthusiasm for universal in-vitro screening of almost 18,000,000 US donors annually.[15(pp16-18),16] More rationally, it favors identification and selective screening of donor populations at increased risk of exposure to infected ticks in endemic areas. Without the robust market created by a universal testing strategy, the manufacturers of assay kits have little economic motive to engage in the expensive research, development, and clinical trials needed to receive a blood donor screening claim from the Food and Drug Administration (FDA). The FDA, without submissions of approvable assays around which to craft guidance, can do little to assist the blood community in controlling the threat.

Trypanosoma cruzi exposes a different facet of the same set of imperatives. Despite fewer than 10 reported transmissions by transfusion in the United States and Canada, representatives of the FDA stated that an acceptable donor screening assay would definitely be followed by a recommendation for its use.[17] With a prospective imprimatur from the regulator, an assay was built and licensed. The blood community adopted, albeit not unanimously, an essentially universal screening paradigm (in the absence of, but perhaps anticipating, FDA guidance). Unexpectedly, early look-back studies suggest that very few transmissions are being prevented despite an astonishing investment.[18] The direct cost of this activity is estimated at more than $100,000,000 annually.

Based on available data about the performance of systems in development, it is arguable that neither developing an assay for infection with *Babesia sp.* nor implementation of *T. cruzi* serology would be needed in the face of PI. Similarly, malaria deferrals for travel to or residence in endemic areas ought to be reconsidered after implementation of a well-validated PI process for red-cell-containing components. The FDA has estimated malaria deferrals cost the US blood community more than 150,000 donors annually and more than 730,000 when considering self-deferrals.[19] Not only are these donors lost for the duration of their deferral, but many never return for future donations even when otherwise fully qualified.

Viruses

Few repeatedly reactive screening tests for human T-cell lymphotropic virus, types I and II, in contemporary US blood donors reflect infection with one of these viruses based on unlicensed confirmatory testing.[20] Both of the donor screening tests that have been used in dual enzyme immunoassay donor retention and counseling strategies have now been withdrawn from the market. The blood community is screening using a single platform, and there will be nothing available to offer reactive donors to help maintain their eligibility or to requalify them after clearly false-positive test results.[21] This leads to thousands of complicated donor counseling sessions annually, and those donors may rightfully question the credibility of the blood community in the face of mixed messages that combine indefinite deferral with assurance that their test results are medically irrelevant. Can a robust PI process for cellular blood components replace serologic testing or at least replace universal serologic screening with a one-time testing approach, as is used in some EU countries?[22] That would mitigate at least some of the impact of using relatively nonspecific assays on donors repeatedly. Would multiple assays for hepatitis B virus [HBV; ie, antibodies to HBV core antigen and HBV surface antigen, with or without HBV nucleic acid testing (NAT)] or HIV and HCV (serology and NAT) still be required in the face of robust PI?

Syphilis

The last alleged case of transfusion-transmitted syphilis in the United States was in the late 1960s. Since that time, rates of primary and secondary syphilis have fallen to historically low levels, but testing continues for infection with *Treponema pallidum* using assays that either are nonspecific, yielding high false-positive rates, or detect the immunologic scar of remote syphilis much more frequently than transfusion-transmissible early infections. Some have argued the serologic test for syphilis is a useful surrogate for behaviors associated with the risk of other recognized transfusion-transmitted infections, but this appears not to be true.[23] Can we stop using the serologic test for syphilis, with its apparent lack of a safety increment and nonspecificity, after implementation of effective PI systems?

Summary

The current transfusion safety paradigm is to await emergence and identification of a transfusion-transmitted agent before responding. Then, when its epidemiology is beginning to be understood, donor history questions and deferral criteria are developed to protect the blood supply. Finally, laboratory tests are built. Ahead of and during these intervals after recognition but before deployment of sensitive and specific donor screening assays, morbidity and mortality accumulate in transfusion recipients. These gaps have been 30 and 15 years, respectively, for serum hepatitis/HBV and posttransfusion non-A,non-B/HCV and more than 3 years for HIV.[24] More recently, with the development of high-throughput NAT for HIV and HCV, then for West Nile virus (WNV), widespread test implementation under FDA investigational new drug exemptions was permitted until sufficient data were acquired to support approval of biologics license applications.

Viewed against this history, the overwhelmingly attractive prospect of PI is *proactivity*—its ability to address agents that behave like those with which we have historically contended and to protect recipients from known, emerging, and even still unrecognized threats. The opportunity for PI is to replace the ascending spiral of donor history deferrals and in-vitro assays for demonstrated, emerging infectious and putative risks with preemption. In the interval between reporting of the first case of transfusion-transmitted WNV infection and the start of testing in the summer of 2003, there were 23 recognized cases.[25] Given passive surveillance and the high ratio of asymptomatic-to-clinical cases seen with vectorial transmission, there were likely many more infections associated with transfusion. During successive seasons, the blood community has gone to great lengths to develop and implement strategies for conversion from minipool NAT to individual donation testing to minimize transmissions from missed low-level viremic donors during seasonal peaks of transmission.[26] Had PI been in use, would an emergency program have been needed to develop, install, and implement and then revise WNV NAT strategies, or would the activity of PI on WNV or model viruses have been validated, resulting in confidence in the safety of the blood supply before infections occurred? Source plasma collectors did not have to implement screening for WNV because the plasma industry uses robust pathogen-inactivation technologies that are highly effective against lipid-enveloped viruses.[27]

Graft-vs-Host Disease

Lethal TA-GVHD is prevented using gamma or X-irradiation of cellular blood products administered to certain patients with cellular immune deficiency and to recipients of units from donors likely to have substantial HLA homology (HLA-matched products, those from close relatives or from donors in genetically homogeneous populations). During 2006 in the United States, 10.3% of cellular products were irradiated (2,322,000 components).[15(p28)] Radiation adversely affects the quality of cellular components, shortening the outdate of Red Blood Cells, and costs on average $50 to $60 per unit in the United States. Also, in the United States it is performed mainly using cesium-137 sources that have recently provoked security concerns.[28] Data demonstrating prevention of GVHD in animal models[29,30] suggest PI can replace the use of radiation in this indication. Clinical trials have been conducted in the EU during which PI replaced gamma irradiation, and no clinical issues were observed.[31,32] Gamma irradiation prophylaxis (and also cytomegalovirus serology and bacterial culture) is being replaced in the EU in some centers that have adopted the Intercept Blood System (Cerus, Concord, CA) for platelets, with no reports to date of TA-GVHD.[33-35] Although the number of patients followed remains small relative to the low incidence of recognized TA-GVHD, this experience suggests PI may be able to replace component irradiation. If applied universally, PI would preempt the need for clinicians to recognize those recipients with risk for TA-GVHD and specifically request irradiated blood.

Regulatory Status

Basic Concerns with the Current Paradigm

PI processes are approved for use with plasma and platelets in the EU. In the United States and Canada, regulatory evaluation and approval is proceeding quite slowly. The most commonly cited concerns include the following[36]:

- With the current high level of safety *from recognized pathogens* in the North American blood supply, the incremental risk/benefit equation of PI remains unacceptable for transfusion recipients.
- The operational complexities and costs of candidate systems, and those inherent in the absence of a single process applicable to whole blood and each of its components, makes implementation impractical.
- Candidate technologies have limitations for inactivating some intrinsically resistant agents [such as parvovirus B19, hepatitis A virus (HAV), and the transmissible spongiform encephalopathy agents] and agents present at spectacularly high titer (such as parvovirus B19 or HBV), and they have limitations from interference with inactivation related to storage-container geometry, interfering substances, or process failures; consequently, they will not be perfect solutions.
- The individual candidate chemicals and their metabolites and photoproducts require evaluation in complex clinical trials for a variety of effects. These include survival, recovery, and function of the therapeutic product as well as acute and chronic adverse effects on recipients (including uniquely vulnerable populations such as neonates and pregnant women), collection facility personnel, and the environment.

The inescapable irony is that the precautionism driving the current defer-and-test strategies is also a brake on the evaluation and approval of PI processes. Implementing any strategy that manipulates blood or plasma, with their current levels of safety from infection, is a risk/benefit exercise for which critical analytic inputs—quantitative risk approximations and estimates of clinical severity and susceptibility to PI of future agents of transfusion-transmitted infection—are missing. The tension between theoretical risks and potential benefits has nearly paralyzed progress in clinical and regulatory evaluation. The following statement by J. Vostal from a consensus conference[37(pp18-20)] recapitulates the dilemma:

> *In summary, the FDA's current perspective on regulation of PI processes requires defining pathogen reduction capacity, the loss of transfusion product efficacy post-PI treatment, the toxicity and adverse event rate in both preclinical and clinical trials, and the current risks of transfusion-transmitted diseases, so that*

a risk-benefit balance of PI processes can be determined. If the risk-benefit balance is favorable, then PI processes would be approved with provisions to limit their use based on transfusion product efficacy, with a request for phase 4 postmarketing studies for adverse event monitoring. If the risk-benefit is deemed unfavorable, approval could be considered in situations where the transfusion-transmitted disease risk would be increased, as in a case of an emerging pathogen epidemic.

Assuming an emerging pathogen will be susceptible to PI, as are the most important known agents, this regulatory calculus, focused as it is on *current risks,* does not try to integrate the *probability* that new "situations where the transfusion-transmitted disease risk would be increased, as in a case of an emerging pathogen epidemic," will undoubtedly arise and ignores the range of morbid outcomes from a new agent and the incidence of transfusion transmissions that would likely occur while an epidemic evolves.

Perspectives on Future Risks

Are future epidemics of transfusion-transmitted infection inevitable?[24] If the answer is yes, how morbid will they be, and can we recognize them more rapidly now than in the early 1980s when HIV entered the blood supply? Can we shorten or avoid the interval during which transfusion will infect recipients before we devise effective interventions? Are there current transfusion-transmissible infections for which effective mitigation strategies are not available? AABB's Transfusion-Transmitted Diseases (TTD) Committee has recently reviewed a long list of known human pathogens and tried to rank them as to their potential to become important TTDs.[38] Sixty-eight agents were selected for analysis in the *TRANSFUSION* supplement article. Seven of eight agents in the highest priority levels (dengue virus, *Babesia sp.*, chikungunya virus, St Louis encephalitis virus, *Leishmania sp., Plasmodium sp.,* and *T. cruzi*), not to mention bacterial contamination of platelets, should be mitigated using the PI processes being developed for cellular blood components and transfusable plasma today. Only the variant Creutzfeldt-Jakob disease (vCJD) prion would not be. Other important pathogens that were not given the highest threat assessment may be poised to breach the safety nets in the future—eg, evolving variants of HIV,

HBV, and WNV that might escape detection with current serologic and/or NAT assays before being recognized.

Two months following publication of the supplement, investigators described a cell-associated gammaretrovirus (XMRV) present in blood, associated with prostate cancer and chronic fatigue syndrome and found in 3.7% of normal controls.[39] Editorialists immediately wondered about blood-borne transmission,[40] and one of the authors began to speculate, in the popular media, on the need to intervene for transfusion safety.[41] In December 2009, the FDA sponsored a workshop titled "Emerging Arboviruses: Evaluating the Threat to Transfusion and Transplantation Safety." At that meeting, more than 500 arbovirus species were recognized, with more than 100 known to infect humans, virtually all with a viremic interval.[42] Their ability to move rapidly around the world and cause severe disease is exemplified by WNV and chikungunya virus. The week of that workshop, severe encephalitis from Usutu virus, a mosquito-borne arbovirus from the Japanese encephalitis group that is known to circulate in European birds but not recognized as an important human pathogen, was reported in a liver transplant recipient in Italy.[43]

Feasibility

Each candidate PI process is indeed fairly complex, but there are no steps that are inconsistent with tasks already performed in blood centers. The facility and personnel requirements sufficient to support the wide range of centers in North America are not completely understood, but the successful implementation and use of PI in the EU and the rapid introduction of PI for plateletpheresis in response to the Réunion Island chikungunya epidemic[44] demonstrate feasibility and compatibility with a good manufacturing practice environment. Blood community concerns about these operational issues must not become code for inertia based on costs.

The absence of a single process that works for all components is certainly not ideal, but it ought not to prevent the application of a workable process to the problem, for example, of bacterial contamination in platelets, with the advantages of more robust systems to be accrued over time. The Canadian Consensus Conference recommended that "until this idealized multicomponent system is a reality, existing pathogen reduction technologies should be implemented for platelets and transfusable plasma, an approach already undertaken in many parts of Europe."[37(p4)]

There are transfusion-transmitted agents that will be relatively resistant to PI by virtue of titer (parvovirus B19 and HBV), the agent's physical characteristics [parvovirus B19, HAV, and transmissible spongiform encephalopathy (TSE) agents], or the mode of action of the PI process (TSE agents). It is conceivable that the next epidemic TTD will be from a resistant agent, but those for which testing and deferral are already required, except TSEs, appear sensitive to the nucleic-acid-based processes being developed. (All of the agents listed as highest-priority agents by the AABB TTD Committee appear to be so.) What is the logic of waiting for approaches that address historically minor but resistant pathogens or those for which there may be no feasible physical process compatible with transfusable components, holding in abeyance methods active against the broad range of the most prevalent current and disconcerting potential targets? The critical implication of potential resistance to inactivation is that vigilance for TTDs, and especially new threats, cannot be reduced in the face of PI, but Voltaire was likely correct: "the best is the enemy of the good."

Risk vs Benefit

The cogent argument for the hindered movement of pathogen reduction systems through the regulatory system is that a risk/benefit advantage has not been established. In an attempt to ensure that toxicologic risks have been minimized, systems to ensure removal of the active PI compounds below levels of detection have been incorporated in some PI systems, and cell culture, animal, and clinical evidence suggest that carcinogenicity, mutagenicity, and acute or chronic toxicity are so low that they are unlikely to annul even the "limited" benefit of a system or systems applied to only platelets to address bacterial contamination. Such an implementation of PI in the United States would mitigate a major cause of transfusion morbidity and of transfusion fatalities reported to the FDA in recent years (transfusion-associated bacterial sepsis), eliminate the need to inoculate and incubate platelet cultures before release, and circumvent consideration of adding near-release rapid bacterial testing to interdict residual episodes of bacterial sepsis. It may be possible to extend the outdate back to 7 days or beyond using PI with platelet additive solutions. This could expand the availability of the product without a need to find more donors—a benefit by itself—but also may enhance the ability to provide TRALI-safe platelets by moving toward male donors or donors lacking antibodies implicated in TRALI pathogenesis. Will confirmation of these benefits compensate for the lower platelet survival and recovery that result from PI processing?

The opinions expressed by members of the FDA's Blood Products Advisory Committee (BPAC) at the November 2009 meeting were an example of stringent precautionism and its potential impact on the willingness and/or ability of sponsors to bring PI systems forward.[45] The SPRINT trial demonstrated noninferiority of amotosalen-treated apheresis platelets for the primary hemostatic endpoint of (World Health Organization) Grade 2 bleeding,[46] but the FDA was concerned about other secondary hemostatic endpoints (eg, days of Grade 2 bleeding, corrected count increments, numbers of platelet transfusions, and days between transfusions). Most important, the FDA was very concerned about a statistically significant excess of serious pulmonary morbidity (acute lung injury and respiratory distress syndrome) in the treatment arm.[47] Overall mortality was statistically equivalent in treatment and control arms of SPRINT. A fairly rigorous blinded retrospective reanalysis of pulmonary reactions performed for the manufacturer by independent experts[48] suggested a less marked and statistically insignificant difference in respiratory adverse events between treatment and control groups. Nevertheless, and appropriately, the study sponsor agreed with the FDA's request for a second Phase III randomized, blinded, controlled trial involving 1024 patients using more conservative hemostatic outcomes and improved monitoring for adverse pulmonary (and other) events.[49] The FDA and the sponsor presented the draft trial design to the advisory committee. Unfortunately, BPAC focused on statistical issues, rejected the proposed trial design, and recommended an alternate study design approximately three times larger (around 3000 patients). In addition, the committee recommended that, even if the second Phase III trial were successful, Phase IV postmarket surveillance for the incidence of acute lung injury should be required as a blinded, randomized controlled trial in a limited number of sites. This unusually rigorous design for the Phase IV postmarketing study seemed to require duplication, inappropriately to some observers, of the proposed pivotal Phase III trial even before results were available. It is unclear whether the sponsor has the resources and is willing to proceed with these two extremely expensive trials. Finally, there was no extended discussion of how to integrate consideration of the risks to the blood supply from emerging infections into the decision-making process, other than a plea by Harvey Alter, MD, from the National Institutes of Health that the committee be cognizant of these potential threats and consider the contribution to safety provided by the proactive approach of PI.

Caution from regulators asked to approve a new process for PI is understandable and necessary. That caution must not be excessive, however, and unconfirmed side effects ought not to make approval in the United States impossible. Those risks need to be analyzed within the context of the seriousness of existing *and future* infections that may be transmitted unwittingly to transfusion recipients. Contemporary PI technologies for cellular components are not perfect, but they have a reassuring safety record in the EU (even recognizing criticisms about the vigor of surveillance).[47] It is interesting to reflect on the impact that a collective memory of HIV in the blood supply had on decisions made around vCJD in the late 1990s.[50] The urgency that regulators, their advisors, and advocacy groups felt about the theoretical transmission of vCJD owed much to the HIV experience. That has led to the deferral of hundreds of thousands of individuals who resided for as little as 3 months in the United Kingdom. This interest in preemptive strategies seems to have waned despite our increasing awareness of emerging infectious diseases[38] that may be transfusion transmissible and the initially favorable evidence about the clinical safety or toxicology of PI.[33,46,48,51-53]

Conclusion

Continued development of a preemptive PI strategy addressing transfusion-transmitted infection is fundamentally a business proposition. Success depends on a strong sense by developers that there is opportunity for regulatory approval and subsequent broad application of the technology. The regulators' task is to balance potential benefits from PI with risks from toxicity and changes in the clinical performance of treated components. Balance is the path to a degree of safety for whole blood and cellular components that approaches that achieved by manufacturers of plasma derivatives in the 1980s. It is at our peril that we ignore future threats in our calculations, deciding that blood products are safe enough. History suggests that may not be the case.

References

1. Busch MP, Young MJ, Samson SM, et al. Risk of human immunodeficiency virus (HIV) transmission by blood transfusions before the implementation of HIV-1 antibody screening. The Transfusion Safety Study Group. Transfusion 1991;31:4-11.
2. Food and Drug Administration. Fatalities reported to FDA following blood collection and transfusion. Rockville, MD: CBER Office of Compliance and Biologics Quality, 2009. [Available at http://www.fda.gov/BiologicsBlood Vaccines/SafetyAvailability/ReportaProblem/TransfusionDonationFatalities/ ucm118316.htm (accessed May 18, 2010).]
3. AuBuchon JP, Cooper LK, Leach MF, et al. Experience with universal bacterial culturing to detect contamination of apheresis platelet units in a hospital transfusion service. Transfusion 2002;42:855-61.
4. Dodd RY. Bacterial contamination and transfusion safety: Experience in the United States. Transfus Clin Biol 2003;10:6-9.
5. Ness P, Braine H, King K, et al. Single-donor platelets reduce the risk of septic platelet transfusion reactions. Transfusion 2001;41:857-61.
6. Brecher ME, Hay SN. Bacterial contamination of blood components. Clin Microbiol Rev 2005;18:195-204.
7. Benjamin RJ, Wagner SJ. The residual risk of sepsis: Modeling the effect of concentration on bacterial detection in two-bottle culture systems and an estimation of false-negative culture rates. Transfusion 2007;47:1381-9.
8. Murphy WG, Foley M, Doherty C, et al. Screening platelet concentrates for bacterial contamination: Low numbers of bacteria and slow growth in contaminated units mandate an alternative approach to product safety. Vox Sang 2008;95:13-19.
9. Dumont LJ, Kleinman S, Murphy JR, et al. Screening of single-donor apheresis platelets for bacterial contamination: The PASSPORT study results. Transfusion 2010;50:589-99.
10. Kleinman S, Dumont L, Tomasulo P, et al. The impact of discontinuation of 7-day storage of apheresis platelets (PASSPORT) on recipient safety: An illustration of the need for proper risk assessments. Transfusion 2009;49:903-12.
11. Picker SM, Oustianskaia L, Schneider V, Gathof BS. Functional characteristics of apheresis-derived platelets treated with ultraviolet light combined with either amotosalen-HCl (S-59) or riboflavin (vitamin B_2) for pathogen-reduction. Vox Sang 2009;97:26-33.
12. Fitzpatrick JEP, Kennedy CC, McGeown MG, et al. Human case of piroplasmosis (babesiosis). Nature 1968;217:861-2.
13. Gubernot DM, Lucey CT, Lee KC, et al. Babesia infection through blood transfusions: Reports received by the US Food and Drug Administration, 1997-2007. Clin Infect Dis 2009;48:25-30.

14. Leiby DA, Chung APS, Cable RG, et al. Relationship between tick bites and the seroprevalence of *Babesia microti* and *Anaplasma phagocytophila* (previously *Ehrlichia sp.*) in blood donors. Transfusion 2002;42:1585-91.
15. The 2007 national blood collection and utilization survey report. Washington, DC: Department of Health and Human Services, 2008.
16. Cable R. In: Food and Drug Administration. Workshop to consider approaches to reduce the risk of transfusion-transmitted babesiosis in the United States (Bethesda, MD, September 12, 2008). Rockville, MD: CBER Office of Communication, Outreach, and Development, 2008. [Available at http://www.fda.gov/BiologicsBloodVaccines/NewsEvents/WorkshopsMeetings Conferences/TranscriptsMinutes/default.htm (accessed May 18, 2010).]
17. Nakhasi H. In: Food and Drug Administration. Transcript of the Blood Products Advisory Committee meeting, September 12, 2002. Rockville, MD: CBER Office of Communication, Outreach, and Development, 2002:291. [Available at http://www.fda.gov/ohrms/dockets/ac/cber02.htm#BloodProd ucts (accessed May 18, 2010).]
18. Food and Drug Administration. Advisory committees. April 1-2, 2009: Briefing information for Blood Products Advisory Committee meeting. Rockville, MD: CBER Office of Communication, Outreach, and Development, 2009. [Available at http://www.fda.gov/AdvisoryCommittees/CommitteesMeeting Materials/BloodVaccinesandOtherBiologics/BloodProductsAdvisoryCommit tee/ucm155529.htm (accessed May 18, 2010).]
19. Anderson S. Risks versus benefits related to the possible implementation of a malaria blood-screening test. FDA workshop on testing for malarial infections in blood donors (July 12, 2006). Rockville, MD: CBER Office of Communication, Outreach, and Development, 2006. [Available at http://www.fda.gov/BiologicsBloodVaccines/NewsEvents/WorkshopsMeetingsConferences/ucm091248.htm (accessed May 18, 2010).]
20. Abbott Diagnostics Division. Package insert. Abbott PRISM HTLV-I/HTLV-II. Abbott Park, IL: Abbott Laboratories, 2007. [Available at http://www.fda.gov/BiologicsBloodVaccines/BloodBloodProducts/ApprovedProducts/Licensed ProductsBLAs/BloodDonorScreening/InfectiousDisease/ucm090707.htm (accessed May 18, 2010).]
21. Food and Drug Administration. Guidance for industry: Donor screening for antibodies to HTLV-II (August 1997). Rockville, MD: CBER Office of Communication, Outreach, and Development, 1997. [Available at http://www.fda.gov/downloads/BiologicsBloodVaccines/GuidanceComplianceRegulatory Information/Guidances/Blood/UCM170916.pdf (accessed May 18, 2010).]
22. Laperche S, Worms B, Pillonel J. European Network of Transfusion Medicine Societies; Steering Committee. Blood safety strategies for human T-cell lymphotropic virus in Europe. Vox Sang 2009;96:104-10.
23. Zou S, Notari EP, Fang CT, et al. Current value of serologic test for syphilis as a surrogate marker for blood borne viral infections among blood donors in the United States. Transfusion 2009;49:636-47.
24. Alter H. Pathogen reduction: A precautionary principle paradigm. Trans Med Rev 2008;22:97-102.

25. Pealer LN, Marfin AA, Petersen LR, et al for the West Nile Virus Transmission Investigation Team. Transmission of West Nile virus through blood transfusion in the United States in 2002. N Engl J Med 2003;349:1236-45.
26. Biggerstaff BJ, Petersen LR. A modeling framework for evaluation and comparison of trigger strategies for switching from minipool to individual-donation testing for West Nile virus. Transfusion 2009;49:1151-9.
27. Food and Drug Administration. Guidance for industry: Assessing donor suitability and blood and blood product safety in cases of known or suspected West Nile virus infection (June 2005). Rockville, MD: CBER Office of Communication, Outreach, and Development, 2005. [Available at http://www.fda.gov/downloads/BiologicsBloodVaccines/GuidanceComplianceRegulatoryInformation/Guidances/Blood/ucm080286.pdf (accessed May 18, 2010).]
28. United States Nuclear Regulatory Commission. SECY-08-0184. Strategy for the security and use of cesium-137 chloride sources (November 24, 2008). Washington, DC: US NRC, 2008. [Available at http://www.nrc.gov/reading-rm/doc-collections/commission/secys/2008/secy2008-0184/2008-0184scy.html (accessed May 18, 2010).]
29. Grass JA, Wafa T, Reames A, et al. Prevention of transfusion-associated graft-versus-host disease by photochemical treatment. Blood 1999;93:3140-7.
30. Fast LD, DiLeone G, Cardarelli G, et al. Mirasol PRT treatment of donor white blood cells prevents the development of xenogeneic graft-versus-host disease in Rag2$^{-/-}$ gamma c$^{-/-}$ double knockout mice. Transfusion 2006;46:1553-60.
31. Schlenke P, Hagenah W, Andresen S, et al. Platelet components treated with pathogen inactivation using the INTERCEPT Blood System: Clinical outcomes of the first single-centre clinical trial in Germany. Vox Sang 2007;93 (Suppl 1):171.
32. Infanti L, Job S, Santoro M, et al. Platelet components treated with pathogen inactivation using the INTERCEPT Blood System: Clinical outcomes of the first single-centre observational trial in Switzerland. Vox Sang 2008;95(Suppl 1):289.
33. Osselaer JC, Cazenave JP, Lambermont M, et al. An active haemovigilance programme characterizing the safety profile of 7437 platelet transfusions prepared with amotosalen photochemical treatment. Vox Sang 2008;94:315-23.
34. Rasonglès P, Angelini-Tibert MF, Simon P, et al. Transfusion of platelet components prepared with photochemical pathogen inactivation treatment during a Chikungunya virus epidemic in Ile de La Réunion. Transfusion 2009;49:1083-91.
35. Osselaer JC, Doyen C, Defoin L, et al. Universal adoption of pathogen inactivation of platelet components: Impact on platelet and red blood cell component use. Transfusion 2009;49:1412-22.
36. Epstein JS, Vostal JG. FDA approach to evaluation of pathogen reduction technology. Transfusion 2003;43:1347-50.
37. Vostal J. In: Weibert KE, Cserti CM, Hannon J, et al. Proceedings of a consensus conference: Pathogen inactivation—making decisions about new technologies. Trans Med Rev 2008;1:1-34.

38. Stramer SL, Hollinger FB, Katz LM, et al. Emerging infectious disease agents and their potential threat to transfusion safety. Transfusion 2009;49(Suppl 2):1S-29S.
39. Lombardi VC, Ruscetti FW, Gupta JD, et al. Detection of an infectious retrovirus, XMRV, in blood cells of patients with chronic fatigue syndrome. Science 2009;326:585-9.
40. Coffin JM, Stoye JP. Perspectives: A new virus for old diseases? Science 2009;326:530-1.
41. Hall J. Chronic fatigue "a true human infection," study says. The Toronto Star, October 9, 2009. [Available at http://www.thestar.com/article/707715 (accessed May 18, 2010).]
42. Food and Drug Administration. Emerging arboviruses: Evaluating the threat to transfusion and transplantation safety. Agenda for public workshop, Bethesda, MD, December 14-15, 2009. Rockville, MD: CBER Office of Communication, Outreach, and Development, 2009. [Available at http://www.fda.gov/downloads/BiologicsBloodVaccines/NewsEvents/WorkshopsMeetingsConferences/UCM193495.pdf (accessed May 18, 2010).]
43. Cavrini F, Gaibani P, Longo G, et al. Rapid communications: Usutu virus infection in a patient who underwent orthotropic liver transplantation, Italy, August-September 2009. Eurosurveillance 2009 (17 December);14:1-2. [Available at http://www.eurosurveillance.org/ViewArticle.aspx?ArticleId=19448 (accessed May 18, 2010).]
44. Rasonglès P, Angelini-Tibert MF, Simon P, et al. Transfusion of platelet components prepared with photochemical pathogen inactivation treatment during a chikungunya virus epidemic in Ile de La Réunion. Transfusion 2009; 49:1083-91.
45. Food and Drug Administration. Transcript of the Blood Products Advisory Committee meeting, Bethesda, MD, November 16, 2009. Topic II: Study designs (Phases 3 and 4) for product development of human platelets using the Cerus INTERCEPT Blood System for pathogen inactivation. Rockville, MD: CBER Office of Communication, Outreach, and Development, 2009:158-361. [Available at http://www.fda.gov/downloads/AdvisoryCommittees/CommitteesMeetingMaterials/BloodVaccinesandOtherBiologics/BloodProductsAdvisoryCommittee/UCM193385.pdf (accessed May 18, 2010).]
46. McCullough J, Vesole DH, Benjamin RJ, et al. Therapeutic efficacy and safety of platelets treated with a photochemical process for pathogen inactivation: The SPRINT Trial. Blood 2004;104:1534-41.
47. Food and Drug Administration. Blood Products Advisory Committee 96th meeting, November 16-17, 2009. Issue summary. Topic II: Study designs (Phases 3 and 4) for product development of human platelets using the Cerus INTERCEPT Blood System for pathogen inactivation. Rockville, MD: CBER Office of Communication, Outreach, and Development, 2009. [Available at http://www.fda.gov/downloads/AdvisoryCommittees/CommitteesMeetingMaterials/BloodVaccinesandOtherBiologics/BloodProductsAdvisoryCommittee/UCM190168.pdf (accessed May 18, 2010).]
48. Snyder E, McCullough J, Slichter SJ, et al. Clinical safety of platelets photochemically treated with amotosalen HCl and ultraviolet A light for pathogen inactivation: The SPRINT trial. Transfusion 2005;45:1864-75.

49. Cerus Corporation. A Phase 3 prospective, randomized, double-blinded, multicenter clinical trial to determine effectiveness and safety of platelet components prepared by photochemical treatment compared to conventional component processes. Briefing material: Blood Products Advisory Committee meeting, November 2009. Concord, CA: Cerus, 2009. [Available at http://www.fda.gov/downloads/AdvisoryCommittees/CommitteesMeetingMaterials/BloodVaccinesandOtherBiologics/BloodProductsAdvisoryCommittee/UCM189568.pdf (accessed May 18, 2010).]
50. Ponte ML. Insights into the management of emerging infections: Regulating variant Creutzfeldt-Jakob disease transfusion risk in the UK and the US (review). PLoS Med. 2006;3(10):e342.
51. Osselaer JC, Messe N, Hervig T, et al. A prospective observational cohort safety study of 5106 platelet transfusions with components prepared with photochemical pathogen inactivation treatment. Transfusion 2008;48:1061-71.
52. Reddy HL, Dayan AD, Cavagnaro J, et al. Toxicity testing of a novel riboflavin-based technology for pathogen reduction and white blood cell inactivation. Transfus Med Rev 2008;22:133-53.
53. Janetzko K, Cazenave JP, Kluter H, et al. Therapeutic efficacy and safety of photochemically treated apheresis platelets processed with an optimized integrated set. Transfusion 2005;45:1443-52.

In: AuBuchon JP, Prowse CV, eds.
Pathogen Inactivation: The Penultimate Paradigm Shift
Bethesda, MD: AABB Press, 2010

17

European Perspectives on Implementation

ERHARD SEIFRIED, MD, PHD;
REINHARD HENSCHLER, MD, PHD; AND
MARKUS M. MUELLER, MD

THIS CHAPTER SUMMARIZES PERSPECTIVES REGARDING pathogen inactivation (PI) from different European blood transfusion services. As one might expect, individual opinions on the topic vary widely. In addition to the scientific issues, the chapter also addresses regulatory and economic aspects of PI in Europe.

Erhard Seifried, MD, PhD, Professor of Transfusion Medicine and Executive Director; Reinhard Henschler, MD, PhD, Head, Research and Development, and Head, Production Department; and Markus M. Mueller, MD, Consultant in Transfusion Medicine, Hemostaseology; Institute for Transfusion Medicine and Immunohematology, Clinics of the Johann Wolfgang Goethe University—Frankfurt/Main, and the German Red Cross Blood Transfusion Service—Baden-Wuerttemberg-Hessen, Frankfurt/Main, Germany

E. Seifried has disclosed no conflicts of interest. R. Henschler and M. Mueller have disclosed financial relationships with Cerus.

The Current Situation in Europe

Blood components for transfusion are classified differently by the various European countries. In Germany, they are considered pharmaceutical drugs, while in other European countries with similarly stringent rules, they are classified as medicinal products. European community (EC) directives such as European Blood Directive 2002/98/EC and all subsequent related directives define quality and safety standards for the collection, testing, processing, storage, and distribution of human blood and blood components.

Individual EC member states are free to adopt higher standards than the ones set in the EC directives. In Germany, blood transfusion services are subject to the German drug law, and they are therefore classified as pharmaceutical producers. For the production and distribution of standard blood components such as red blood cells (RBC), platelet concentrates (PC), and fresh frozen plasma (FFP), production licenses issued by local authorities as well as marketing authorizations issued by the competent federal authority are required. Major changes in blood component production therefore require that the transfusion service reapply for a new licence. Similar product approval systems are in place in other countries, eg, France and Switzerland.

Legally binding guidelines imply that pharmaceutical producers have to ensure they apply the latest standards of knowledge in science and technology in their blood products. These quality and safety standards help transfusion services ensure that the blood products they issue meet pharmaceutical standards. Active therapeutic ingredients must be as pure as technically possible, and contaminants must be avoided to the highest degree technically possible under the latest standards of research and development. This led, for example, to the implementation of universal leukocyte reduction at blood component production in most European countries shortly after 2000.

Quality management systems have been continuously improved over the last decade and nowadays have reached the highest industrial standards. Transfusion services have certified quality management systems, and their institutions are often accredited units, like the authors' facility since 2001. Similar quality standards also apply to blood donor selection, donor care, production laboratories, and storage and distribution of blood components as well as clinical consultation by transfusion medicine specialists.

To ensure the lowest residual risk of pathogen contamination of blood products that is technically feasible, regular blood donor screening for all products was established in the 1970s. Between 1970 and 1990, serologic screening was established for syphilis infection and proteins associated with hepatitis B virus (HBV; ie, hepatitis B surface antigen, or HBsAg), immunologic response to HBV infection (antibodies to hepatitis B core antigen, or anti-HBc), hepatitis C virus (anti-HCV), human immunodeficiency virus (anti-HIV-1/2), and cytomegalovirus (anti-CMV). These tests, which have been periodically improved, are helpful in detecting clinically undetectable infections in donors. However, it very soon became clear that a significant "diagnostic window" for some infections remains and that a feasible, economical, and quick method for direct detection of transfusion-transmitted viruses—especially HIV, HCV, and HBV—would be worthwhile. After the HIV disaster at the beginning of the 1980s, European transfusion services concentrated their efforts on further improving the quality and safety of blood donor selection and the testing of blood components for viruses via polymerase chain reaction (PCR) assays. At the authors' facility, for example, nucleic acid testing (NAT) for HIV, HBV, and HCV was introduced in routine blood donor screening for all blood donations in January 1997. This was the first large-scale routine NAT testing that had been implemented for all blood donations.[1]

Today, thanks to the widespread use of HIV and HCV NAT, transfusion-transmitted HIV and HCV infections are very rare. Hourfar et al recently calculated the residual risk of virus transmission by transfusion using data from more than 30 million voluntary blood donations of the Red Cross tested in Germany.[2] The residual risk of HCV transmission by a blood product was estimated to be 1 in 10.88 million transfused units [95% confidence interval (CI): 7.51 to 19.72 million]. For HIV-1, the residual risk was calculated to be 1 in 4.3 million transfused units (95% CI: 2.39 to 21.37 million). For HBV, the results were 1 in 360,000 transfused units (95% CI: 0.19 to 3.36 million). Taking into account the number of blood products transfused in Germany each year—about 4 million RBCs, 400,000 PCs, and 1.1 million packs of FFP (data for the year 2007 from the German federal authority, the Paul Ehrlich Institute[3])—the impact of NAT testing on blood safety has been considerable.

In reality, these results might even be better. Since 1999, when NAT for HCV became mandatory for blood donor screening in Germany, only one case of transfusion-transmitted HCV has been reported, whereas before, cases were reported every year.

Nowadays, the transfusion of blood products is a safe medical procedure, much safer than ever before in the history of medicine. As a result, hitherto underrated risks of hemotherapy have become relatively more prominent. Bacterial contamination of PCs, most often by presumably innocuous residual skin flora coming from donors' deep skin layers, is a rare complication, but in the case of immunocompromised recipients, a potentially dangerous one.

Testing for bacteria in PCs is a cumbersome and expensive technique that currently identifies only about half of the contaminants before the time of transfusion. Hence, novel techniques such as PI methods, especially for PCs, are being considered or are being introduced into blood component production in a number of European countries.

Novel and re-emerging pathogens[4,5] have also been recognized as threats to blood safety. Some may be emerging as a result of global warming and globalization itself, and they require ongoing vigilance to avoid infection disasters via the blood chain (Table 17-1). For almost all of these pathogens, testing is a feasible approach, but the time required to react by implementing specific tests and therefore interdicting transfusion of contaminated units is inherently long. PI, in contrast, can solve these problems proactively.

To obtain a comprehensive overview of the current status of the field of PI in Europe, the authors conducted a survey on testing for pathogens and PI. The survey was sent out via the European Blood Alliance (EBA) network to EBA members in the second half of 2009. Twenty regional and national transfusion services replied, providing information on their current situation, their plans, and their views on PI.

2009 Survey of Pathogen Reduction in Europe

Background

The pathogen reduction status survey consisted of five questions. The first question asked which pathogens were tested for and which

Table 17-1. Emerging or Re-Emerging Pathogens*

Year(s) of Emergence	Pathogen	Transfusion-Transmissible
1980	HTLV-I	Yes
1981	*Borrelia burgdorferi* / Lyme disease	Yes
1981/1982	HTLV-III (HIV-1) / AIDS	Yes
1982	*Escherichia coli* O157:H7	Yes
1982	HTLV-II	Yes
1983	*Helicobacter pylori*	Maybe
1986	*Cyclospora* species	Maybe
1986	HIV-2	Yes
1986	*Ehrlichia* species	Yes
1988	HHV-6	Maybe
1988	Hepatitis E virus (Caliciviridae)	Yes
1989	Hepatitis C virus (Flaviviridae)	Yes
1992	*Vibrio* O 139	Maybe
1992	*Bartonella henselae*	Yes
1993	Sin nombre virus	Maybe
1995	Hepatitis G virus (Flaviviridae)	Yes
1995	HHV-8	Yes
1996	Variant Creutzfeldt-Jakob disease	Yes
1997	Avian influenza virus type A (H5N1)	Maybe
1999	West Nile virus (Flaviviridae) in USA	Yes
1999	Nipah virus	Maybe
2003	SARS (Coronaviridae)	Maybe
2003	Monkeypox virus	Maybe
2004	Metapneumovirus	Maybe
2005	Chikungunya virus in Ile de la Réunion	Yes
2006	Chikungunya virus in France	Yes
2007	Chikungunya virus in Italy	Yes
2008	West Nile virus in Italy and Hungary	Yes
2009	"Swine flu" (influenza A H1N1 virus)	Maybe

*Adapted from Woolhouse[4] and Seifried.[5]
HTLV = human T-cell lymphotropic virus; HHV = human herpes virus; SARS = severe acute respiratory syndrome.

techniques (serology, culture, or NAT) were used. Next, survey participants were asked about which PI methods were being used and the range of blood components on which they were used. Another question dealt with clinical studies in the field of PI—those in the past, currently running protocols, or those planned for the future. Finally, the general attitude of each transfusion service regarding PI as well as specific legal or licensing aspects in implementing PI were assessed.

Survey Results

Detailed responses were received and analyzed from 20 regional and national blood transfusion services in Northern, Eastern, Western, and Southern Europe: Andalusia (Spain), Austria, Belgium (one each from the French-speaking part and the Flemish-speaking part), Denmark, England, Estonia, Finland, France, Germany, Ireland, Italy, Luxembourg, Malta, Portugal, Scotland, Slovenia, Sweden, Switzerland, and Wales. The answers from some regions or countries, such as France for example, apply to the situation in the whole country (the French blood transfusion service is centralized), whereas other blood transfusion services cover and could answer for only parts of the blood supply in their country. Their answers regarding attitude or plans for PI might therefore not reflect the attitude across the whole country.

Testing for Pathogens

Viruses. Of the 20 European transfusion services that responded to the survey, all 20 perform serologic testing for HIV-1/2, HCV, and HBV in compliance with the minimal requirement in European Directive 2002/98/EC.[6] In addition to serology, 18 of 20 centers also perform NAT for HIV-1, 10 use NAT for HIV-2, 16 (80%) perform an HCV PCR test, and 13 use an HBV PCR test (see Fig 17-1).

Testing for hepatitis A virus (HAV) is performed only by five centers, all five using NAT, while one uses a serologic HAV antibody test in addition to NAT. Serologic CMV testing is performed by nine, most of them performing this test only in some regions or on parts of their donations as required for specific groups of patients.

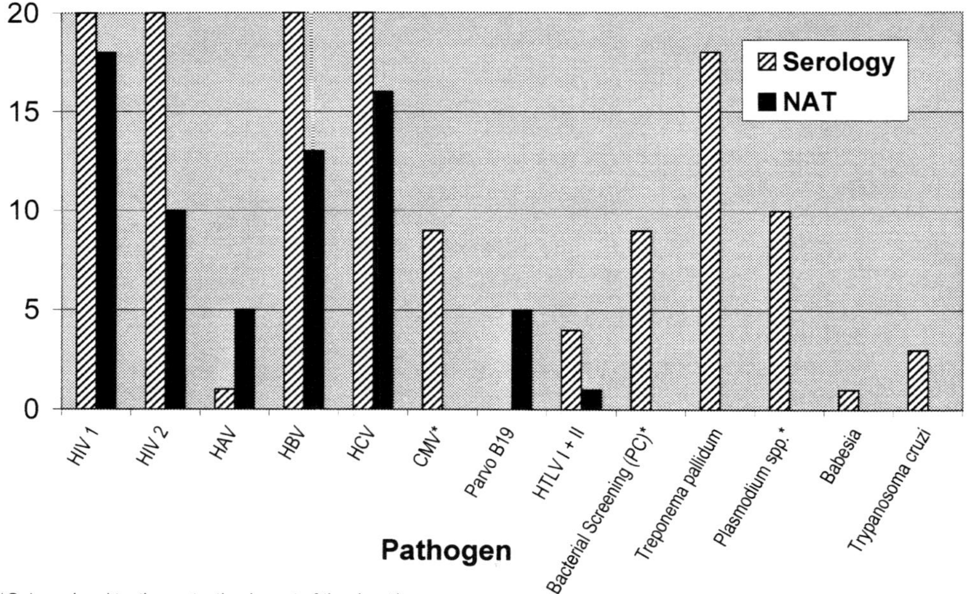

*Only regional testing or testing in part of the donations

Figure 17-1. Number of European blood transfusion services (from a total of 20) testing to detect the indicated pathogen (NAT and/or serology and/or bacterial culture). (Results from the 2009 Survey of Pathogen Reduction in Europe.)
NAT = nucleic acid testing; HIV-1 = human immunodeficiency virus, type 1; HAV = hepatitis A virus; HBV = hepatitis B virus; HCV = hepatitis C virus; CMV = cytomegalovirus; parvo B19 = parvovirus B19; HTLV I + II = human T-cell lymphotropic virus, types I and II; PC = platelet concentrate.

NAT for parvovirus B19 is performed in five, and an additional five (25%) test for human T-cell lymphotropic virus, types I and II. Four of these use a serologic test, while one uses a 48-sample minipool NAT. Tests for West Nile virus and chikungunya virus have been established and validated in one center and can be used if required. Figure 17-1 shows the number of centers testing for various pathogens using serologic tests, NAT, or both for various viruses.

Bacteria. Testing for bacteria by culture, especially in PCs, is performed by nine centers, but some of these test only in a quality control mode or in clinical research studies. Routine testing for bacteria in all products is established in some countries as required by their competent authorities, while it is being considered for implementation in others. Eighteen (90%) perform a test for *Treponema pallidum.*

Protozoa. Ten centers (50%) test for *Plasmodium* species in blood donations. However, some perform this test only on specific donors or in clearly specified cases or situations. One center tests for *Babesia* species, while three test for *Trypanosoma cruzi*, the protozoan causing Chagas disease.

Pathogen Inactivation

Figure 17-2 illustrates the results of the survey according to various aspects of PI described below and in further sections.

Established Techniques. PI is routinely used in 16 of the 20 centers (80%). In 13 of the 16 centers routinely using PI, therapeutic plasma (FFP) is inactivated. In nine of the 13, PI for FFP is performed nationwide, while in five, PI application to FFP varies by locale. The reason that the totals for the breakdown data exceed the number of facilities responding is that in some regions, different PI techniques are used for the same blood component—one technique because of national requirements and others for specific age or disease groups on a local basis. The same holds true for PI for different blood components. Some of the centers using PI for FFP (13/20) also do so for PCs: 8 of the 16 centers using PI (50%) perform PI for PCs, all of them on a local basis. Mandatory introduction of PI for platelets is either under consideration by the respective national competent authorities (as of summer 2009) or strongly recommended by them (two countries).

Methodology Used. For FFP PI, both solvent/detergent (SD) and methylene blue/light (MB) inactivation techniques are frequently used. Nine centers use SD, seven use MB, and two use the amotosalen plus ultraviolet A (UVA) light PI technique for FFP. Again, some centers use more than one PI technique for FFP. The authors' facility has had long-standing experience and has performed studies with both MB and amotosalen/UVA technology for PI of FFP.

PI methods for PCs are more uniform in Europe compared to PI for FFP. Eight centers use amotosalen/UVA; one uses riboflavin/UVB in addition. All PC PI techniques are currently used on a local basis. The authors' facility obtained a production license and marketing authorization for PC PI technology in 2008 but currently uses it in clinical studies or observation programs only. A few centers, eg, in France and Belgium, have lengthy experience with amotosalen/UVA-treated PCs and FFP in routine clinical use.

Plans to Introduce PI in the Future. Ten centers (50%) plan to introduce PI for the first time or to expand their current PI portfolio in the near future. In three countries, this broadening of the PI spectrum (eg, introduction of PI for PCs as well as for FFP, which was introduced in these countries some years ago) has been requested by their competent authority, and it has been strongly recommended in other countries. In more than one country, obligatory introduction of PI for PCs is currently under consideration by the competent authorities. Six of the 10 centers planning to enlarge their PI spectrum or to introduce PI for the first time are doing so without a requirement from their competent authorities.

PI Studies. Ten centers (50%) perform PI studies and are actively involved in the trials or have been so in the past. In addition, four plan to initiate studies or to become active in PI studies in the near future.

Most past, ongoing, or future studies deal with PI for PCs. Facilities involved in PC PI studies have performed or are planning to perform more than one study using either several techniques or PI for PC and FFP. These range from observation programs and hemovigilance studies to randomized, controlled, double-blinded clinical trials. Eight centers have gathered experience with amotosalen/UVA technique for PC PI during these studies, while three have also conducted PC PI studies using riboflavin/UVB. Two further centers are planning to perform studies using amotosalen/UVA technique, and two will perform PC PI studies using riboflavin/UVB.

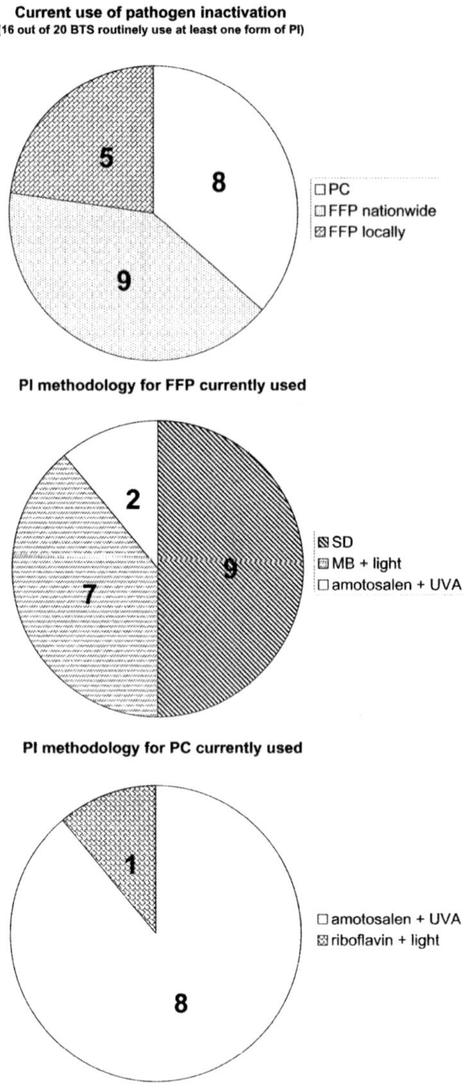

Figure 17-2. Results from the 2009 Survey of Pathogen Reduction in Europe, which surveyed 20 regional and national blood transfusion services across all areas of Europe. Numbers indicate centers according to their responses.
PI = pathogen inactivation; PC = platelet concentrate; FFP = fresh frozen plasma; SD = solvent/detergent; MB = methylene blue; UVA = ultraviolet A (light).

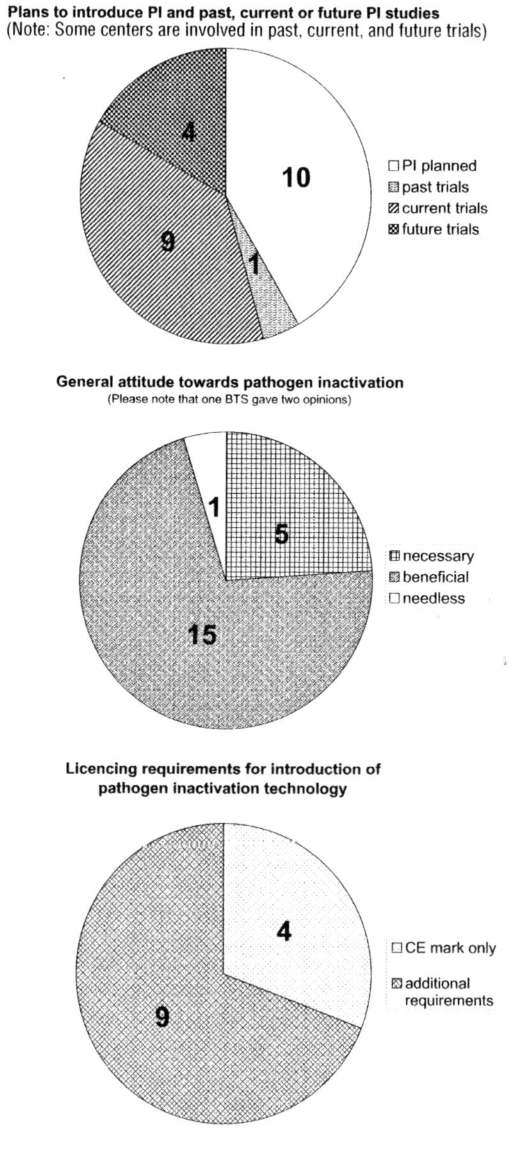

Figure 17-2. (Continued) Results from the 2009 Survey of Pathogen Reduction in Europe, which surveyed 20 regional and national blood transfusion services across all areas of Europe. Numbers indicate centers according to their responses.
PI = pathogen inactivation; CE = Conformité Européenne.

PI studies for FFP have been performed by two centers using the amotosalen/UVA PI technology.

Controlled, randomized, double-blinded clinical trials published earlier have studied the clinical efficacy of pathogen-inactivated PCs from European centers. As one example, results from the euro-SPRITE trial[7] were published in 2003, evaluating the therapeutic efficacy and safety of amotosalen/UVA-treated, buffy-coat-derived PCs vs conventional PCs in 103 thrombocytopenic patients requiring repeated platelet transfusions for up to 56 days. There were no statistically significant differences in the mean 1-hour corrected count increment, clinical hemostasis, and adverse events between the two treatment groups. Patients were enrolled in this trial from the Netherlands, Sweden, the United Kingdom, and France. More recent clinical studies with riboflavin/UVB have also been conducted in Europe.

General Attitude of European Blood Transfusion Services Toward Pathogen Inactivation

Fifteen of 20 centers regard PI as a beneficial technology for further improving the safety of their blood products, and five judge PI technologies as necessary to improve the quality of blood components. Only one judged PI as an unnecessary technology.

However, having stated the beneficial effects of PI for further improvement of safety, some facilities believe that PI should be introduced on a general basis only when "appropriate, safe, and cost-effective technology is available to support implementation" (as stated in one response). Rising production and, therefore, component costs are seen by most centers as a major problem, especially in countries where not-for-profit organizations have limited options for recovering costs by reducing test procedures or simplifying product logistics and stock management. Some facilities that are unable to recover costs using the above-mentioned methods will not be able to implement PI technology because of their current financial situations.

Another issue for most facilities is the loss of procoagulant content or a potential loss in hemostatic efficacy. These concerns have to be viewed in the light of decreasing blood donations and increasing demand for PCs in some countries. Independent (ie, not industry-sponsored), randomized, double-blinded clinical trials with clinically meaningful endpoints that take into account long-term safety and tolerability as well as interactions between drugs have not been performed in a large number of facilities, and thus local data are not available for decision making. In addition, most centers feel that long-term experience with various PI technologies would be helpful before making a final decision.

While acknowledging the benefits of PI in reducing the risks of "pathogens that are unknown, are not tested for, or cannot be avoided" (as stated in one response), some centers would prefer to introduce PI technologies that have proven beyond reasonable doubt that the clinical efficacy of PI blood components is identical to those not treated by PI and that pose no concerns for long-term detrimental effects, side effects, or drug-drug interactions.

Specific Legal Aspects in the Introduction of Pathogen-Inactivation Technology

Thirteen centers (65%) have to submit additional documentation to their competent authorities before introducing PI methods into their production process. However, there are differences in the quality and quantity of documentation required in each country. Some authorities require only that the PI technology be CE (Conformité Européenne) marked, but most other authorities (for nine centers) require submission of additional documents. For example, some centers have to obtain a specific license or permission from their national health authority or an approval from the national pharmaceutical institute or another competent body. Others need both a production license issued by local authorities and a marketing authorization issued by the responsible national authority. The licensing process requires that production, quality control, and in some cases preclinical and clinical data be submitted, not only by the manufacturer of the PI technology but also by the transfusion service.

In some centers, the national requirements depend on the PI methodology to be introduced, while in others, PI is considered a "major modification" of their final blood product, which needs regulatory approval. Still other centers have to change their existing licenses in order to include PI blood products.

In summary, although considerable differences exist among the various European nations in the hurdles to provide PI blood products, nearly 50% of centers have to submit additional documentation to their national authorities and obtain a license and/or authorization to market these products.

Recent and Future Developments

Overall, the European outlook for introducing PI technology in routine blood component production is multifaceted. Regulations vary among European countries, and decision-makers have different scientific, medical, and political viewpoints. In principle, the regulatory framework setting high standards for procuring safe blood in Europe has been established and largely harmonized by European Directive 2002/98/EC, issued by the European Commission and approved by the European Parliament. However, it appears that the health secretary of the European Commission has not yet begun dealing with, discussing, or defining common points on PI technologies, despite the fact that achieving European-wide improvements in supplying safe blood was a major goal of the "Public Health Initiative 2003-2008," launched by the European Commission. No single project in this initiative dealt specifically with creating a common European standpoint or harmonized approach to the implementation of PI.

Problems Commonly Encountered in Implementing Pathogen-Inactivation Technologies

Most European transfusion services consider the introduction of PI technology, especially for PCs, with some reluctance, although the principal benefit of PI is accepted. In countries where PI of blood products has become mandatory (or will soon), such hesitation is over. The remaining European countries, however, revealed different concerns regarding PI technologies for PCs.

First, platelet loss and the potentially reduced hemostatic function as a result of PI are still a matter of debate. Clinical studies with meaningful clinical hemostatic efficacy endpoints comparing equipotent therapeutic doses of PI-treated and non-PI-treated PCs are scarce and almost completely industry driven.

Second, long-term safety regarding some toxicity issues (eg, remaining long-term toxicity or neoantigen formation and, therefore, refractoriness) are still a matter of debate. These concerns may not always be well founded; however, they are still present.

Third, financial resources for introduction and licensing of PI technology are scarce for a substantial number of European transfusion services when the competent authorities refrain from introducing PI as mandatory in their respective countries. Furthermore, not-for-profit organizations in such cases must convince their customers to accept higher blood product costs because they can recover only parts of the cost increment posed by PI technology. As a result of the recent economic crisis, this is quite a task for most centers.

A more general view, encountered in discussions with responsible persons and interested physicians in the field of transfusion medicine in Europe, involves a strong desire to be able to inactivate pathogens in all blood components at the same time and thereby achieve a corresponding increase in the safety of the entire blood supply. This implies PI of RBCs also, not just PCs or FFP. RBC PI research and implementation studies using a chemical, psoralen-based technique is ongoing in several European blood transfusion services, including the authors' facility, as well as in the United States. Moreover, the possibility of inactivating all of a whole blood donation instead of treating each individual component separately is intriguing to many.

Finally, in many European transfusion services, a policy of using at least two suppliers of blood bags or PI systems has been implemented, mainly for reasons of security of the blood supply. However, in the specific case of currently available systems for PI, just to find a second supplier and appropriately license two alternative PI technologies at the same time has been very difficult.

Conclusions

Challenges

Although today's blood components in Europe are safer than ever before, research and development to further improve transfusion safety is a "never ending" and necessary task. Currently, the European debate on reducing pathogen risk can be broken down into two strategies, either testing for pathogens or PI. The benefit of testing is that no drugs have to be added to the products and that it works for all blood components (because testing of the blood donation itself is feasible), but it also has some drawbacks. Testing is restricted to the pathogens one can test for, so unknown or emerging or re-emerging pathogens cannot be detected. Testing leads to a certain delay in release and distribution of blood products, including a time-dependent loss in product quality. Costs for testing, in contrast to PI techniques, depend on the number of pathogens a center has to test for.

PI is also capable of inactivating a broad range of (possibly still unknown) pathogens, including viruses, bacteria, protozoa, and leukocytes. However, none of the currently available methods is effective against all pathogens. Some viruses and bacterial spores, for example, are quite resistant to most PI technologies. There is still no universal routine methodology available for all three standard blood components (RBCs, PCs, and FFP). In addition, each method leads to a loss of activity or active ingredients in the final product compared to non-PI-treated components. Finally, the increase in production costs caused by these novel technologies is substantial and poses a challenge to most European transfusion services, especially not-for-profit organizations that have to raise prices beyond those for standard blood components. Partial cost control can be accomplished by novel approaches to PI technology, such as the authors' approach to pooled, buffy-coat-derived PCs, by which seven buffy coats are pooled and inactivated. The PI-treated PC obtained is then divided into two final products. This approach is currently under evaluation. Another option to control costs might be to reduce the sensitivity of tests, for example by increasing the pool sizes in PCR testing in order to detect only the high viremic donations and using an additional PI method to inactivate the remaining pathogens in donations in which the pathogen level is below the detection limit of the initial test.

Health insurance systems or societies will have to cover increased costs for PI in the end. Current efforts to reduce health-care budgets in most European countries have already led to difficulties and concerns that the blood supply and its quality may come under pressure. This makes it more difficult to think of introducing more cost- and work-intensive methods to blood component production.

There is nonetheless a clear-cut determination in all European transfusion services to fulfil the highest standards and therefore provide the safest blood products possible. This attitude prevails in the vast majority of European countries. Introducing an "ideal" universal PI methodology as described above into routine blood component production is deemed beneficial by almost all centers surveyed in Europe. Some feel that this "ideal" PI is not yet available. At a minimum, most transfusion services in Europe would like independent long-term efficacy and safety studies that meet the highest standards to provide clear clinical data before making a final decision.

Outlook

Novel techniques and methods will increase production costs. Sharp increases in costs can be attenuated by implementing novel rationalization methods in blood component production in some countries. The German Red Cross blood transfusion services were among the first to introduce universal leukocyte reduction and the first to implement NAT for HIV, HCV, and HBV. Nevertheless, overall costs for blood components in Germany are among the lowest in Europe and the Western World. However, some countries feel there could be difficulties in implementing novel costly technologies during the global financial crisis or are doubtful about the cost/benefit tradeoff at this stage. As a result, they are continuing to assess the situation.

Achieving "zero risk" in hemotherapy is an impossible goal but one that society nevertheless demands; therefore, it must be funded accordingly.

Acknowledgments

Most experienced practitioners in European blood transfusion services provided us with information about the current status of testing and PI in their organizations and gave us valuable insights about their views on PI. The authors wish to thank colleagues from Andalusia (Spain), Austria, Belgium (both the French-speaking and Flemish-speaking parts), Denmark, England, Estonia, Finland, France, Germany, Ireland, Italy, Luxembourg, Malta, Portugal, Scotland, Slovenia, Sweden, Switzerland, and Wales for their help.

The logistical help of the European Blood Alliance platform for our 2009 Survey of Pathogen Reduction in Europe is highly appreciated. The authors want to specifically thank Willemijn Kramer for her help. The proofreading by Martina Pfahl is also highly appreciated by the authors.

References

1. Roth WK, Weber M, Seifried E. Feasibility and efficacy of routine PCR screening of blood donations for hepatitis C virus, hepatitis B virus, and HIV-1 in a blood-bank setting. Lancet 1999;353:359-63.
2. Hourfar MK, Jork C, Schottstedt V, et al for the German Red Cross NAT Study Group. Experience of the German Red Cross blood donor services with nucleic acid testing: Results of screening more than 30 million blood donations for human immunodeficiency virus-1, hepatitis C virus and hepatitis B virus. Transfusion 2008;48:1558-66.
3. Henseler O, Heiden M, Haschberger B, et al. Report on notifications pursuant to §21 German Transfusion Act for 2007. Transfus Med Hemother 2010; 37:29-47.
4. Woolhouse MEJ. Population biology of emerging and re-emerging pathogens. Trends Microbiol 2002;10(Suppl):S3-7.
5. Seifried E, Mueller MM. European Parliamentary Public Hearing on "the impact of SARS and other emerging pathogens on transfusion medicine." Blood Therapies in Medicine 2003;3:109-10.
6. Directive 2002/98/EC of the European Parliament and of the Council of 27 January 2003 setting standards of quality and safety for the collection, testing, processing, storage, and distribution of human blood and blood components. Official Journal of the European Union 2003 (8.2.2003);L33/30-40. [Available at http://eur-lex.europa.eu/LexUriServ/LexUriServ.do?uri=OJ:L:2003:033:0030:0040:EN:PDF (accessed May 21, 2010).]
7. van Rhenen D, Gulliksson H, Cazenave JP, et al. Transfusion of pooled buffy coat platelet components prepared with photochemical pathogen inactivation treatment: The euroSPRITE trial. Blood 2003;101:2426-33.

Index

Page numbers in italics indicate tables or figures

G

H

I

N

O

P

S

V

W